HOW TO
RESOLVE THE
HEALTH CARE
CRISIS

How to Resolve the Health Care Crisis

Affordable Protection for All Americans

The Editors of Consumer Reports

CONSUMER REPORTS BOOKS
A Division of Consumers Union
Yonkers, New York

Library of Congress Catalog Card Number: 92-082813
ISBN 0-89043-626-6

Produced by Spectrum America
Design by Constance Baldwin
Charts by Jean Wisenbaugh
First printing, August 1992
Manufactured in the United States of America ♲

How to Resolve the Health Care Crisis is a Consumer Reports Book published by Consumers Union, the nonprofit organization that publishes *Consumer Reports*, the monthly magazine of test reports, product Ratings, and buying guidance. Established in 1936, Consumers Union is chartered under the Not-For-Profit Corporation Law of the State of New York.

The purposes of Consumers Union, as stated in its charter, are to provide consumers with information and counsel on consumer goods and services, to give information on all matters relating to the expenditure of the family income, and to initiate and to cooperate with individual and group efforts seeking to create and maintain decent living standards.

Consumers Union derives its income solely from the sale of *Consumer Reports* and other publications. In addition, expenses of occasional public service efforts may be met, in part, by nonrestrictive, noncommercial contributions, grants, and fees. Consumers Union accepts no advertising or product samples and is not beholden in any way to any commercial interest. Its Ratings and reports are solely for the use of the readers of its publications. Neither the Ratings, nor the reports, nor any Consumers Union publication, including this book, may be used in advertising or for any commercial purpose. Consumers Union will take all steps open to it to prevent such uses of its material, its name, or the name of *Consumer Reports*.

CONTENTS

FOREWORD

The debate over health care reform rages on in America, but it's hard for the average American to find out the facts. Good information is essential if citizens are not to cede the debate to those who are satisfied with things just the way they are, or who would make inconsequential fixes. American consumers need to have certain questions answered.

- How does the present health care system work, and where does it not work?
- Why are health care costs rising so rapidly, and how can they be controlled?
- What level of health care do Americans now have, and what might we expect from a better system?
- How does our system compare with those of other industrialized countries, especially the much discussed, often maligned Canadian system?

To help provide the information that the American public needs to make sense of the debate over health care reform, the editors of *Consumer Reports* have collected in this book the major articles on the U.S. health care system that have appeared in the magazine over the past several years. Written from the perspective of the consumer, these articles range from a dissection of our costly, unfair, and haphazard private health insurance industry to an examination of the strengths (and weaknesses) of the Canadian system. These articles explore the myths promulgated by what Dr. Arnold Relman, the former editor of the *New England Journal of Medicine*, has called the "medical-industrial complex."

Good information can help consumers distinguish between the myths and the facts about health care in America.

Myth: Although some 35 million people are not covered by insurance, the rest of us are getting high-quality care.

Fact: Not all the rest of us are served well. Many are victims of a system that traffics in superfluous equipment, unnecessary and potentially harmful surgery, overmedication, and questionable procedures. Consumers end up paying the ever-escalating bill for all this, either directly or—when employers cut back on coverage—indirectly.

Myth: Our country cannot afford to spend much more to improve health care.

Fact: It doesn't have to. *Consumer Reports* estimates that the combination of waste and excessive administrative costs amounts to $200 billion annually— enough to provide quality care to all Americans without additional government spending.

Myth: Our system provides us the best medical care in the world.

Fact: Our system puts us near the bottom among industrialized countries in infant mortality, in the availability of high-quality primary care, and in public satisfaction.

Myth: Canadians have long waits for heart surgery, and they are dissatisfied with their health care system.

Fact: Canadians have far greater access than people in the United States to all kinds of health care, including heart surgery, and hold their system in the highest esteem.

Myth: A universal, government-financed health system would put a huge, faceless bureaucracy between doctors and their patients.

Fact: The United States already has a huge, costly, intrusive health care bureaucracy—namely, the private insurance companies. Single-payer systems in other countries spend about half what we do on administrative costs and relieve doctors of wasteful, time-consuming paperwork.

The process of researching and analyzing the information presented in this book has led us to formulate our own proposal for health care reform. We believe that the United States needs a health care system based on coverage for everyone, the right to choose your own doctor, and a single payer to control costs. Our proposal is explained in Chapter 7.

If the facts in this book lead you to where they have led us, it's important that your voice be heard by Congress and the Administration. Here's what you can do:

1.   Let members of Congress—and Presidential and Congressional candidates, too—know how much you care, and why. Tell them your experiences. Ask them where they stand on health care reform.

2.   Let them know you want them to vote in *your* interests—not in the interests of the

insurance companies, drug companies, and medical and hospital lobbyists.

3. Let them know that you support a health care system that covers *everyone*, with quality care and with costs controlled effectively through a single payer.

4. Make a commitment to get involved, and stay involved, until we have an American health care system that truly works for all of us. At the back of this book, you will find addresses for members of Congress and a list of ways you can help.

Rhoda H. Karpatkin
Executive Director
Consumers Union of United States, Inc.

INTRODUCTION

This book examines the forces behind the current crisis in health care and looks at possible solutions. In the final chapter we outline the health care reform proposal that Consumers Union favors as providing the best combination of universal access, quality care, and cost containment.

In Chapter 1, "Wasted Health Care Dollars," we explain how the United States manages to spend more money on health care—both per capita and as a percentage of its gross national product—than any other country in the world, and yet fails to provide universal coverage. We show how the "system" that has developed since World War II has enriched providers and insurance companies, channeled unnecessary, too costly, and even harmful treatment to some, and denied the most basic care to others.

In Chapter 2, "The Crisis in Health Insurance," we show how the mainstay of coverage for people under 65—private health insurance—has come to exclude the very people most in need of its protection. We explain how the business practices of insurance companies drive up costs for everyone. For those who must buy individual health insurance, we examine the pitfalls to avoid and the features to insist on.

In Chapter 3, "Is Managed Care the Answer?" we look closely at health maintenance organizations, preferred-provider organizations, and other types of managed care that represent the insurance industry's latest answer to the problem of rising health care costs. We present the results of *Consumer Reports'* first-ever reader survey on HMOs, rate the largest ones, and give advice on selecting managed-care plans.

In Chapter 4, "Health Coverage for Those 65 and Over," we enter the tricky terrain of insurance policies sold to supplement Medicare coverage. We explain recent reforms of these policies and also discuss an alternative form of Medicare: HMOs that serve Medicare recipients.

In Chapter 5, "Long-Term Care Insurance," we expose the duplicitous selling practices and inadequate provisions of coverage for nursing-home care and home care. We show how to decide when such policies are even necessary, and how to select the best of a generally inadequate lot.

In Chapter 6, "Alternative Systems," we visit Canada to see how its citizens like their publicly financed universal system. We compare U.S. and Canadian families with similar health situations, to see how well their respective systems care for them. We also visit Minneapolis, Minnesota, where HMOs dominate the health care landscape more commandingly than in any other place, and Hawaii, which comes closer than any other state to providing universal health coverage.

In Chapter 7, "Time for a Change: Health Coverage for All Americans," we lay out our case for a single-payer system tailored to the needs of the United States. We show how, in our opinion, such a system would solve the problems we have seen and for the first time bring the United States into the company of nations that deliver high-quality, cost-controlled health care to all their citizens as a matter of right.

OUR CURRENT SYSTEM: COSTLY AND EXCLUSIONARY

1
WASTED
HEALTH CARE
DOLLARS

"I can't imagine a system that's more dysfunctional than the one we have now—more expensive, not doing the job, with more waste."

O f the $817 billion that we will spend in 1992 on health care, we will throw away at least $200 billion on overpriced, useless, even harmful treatments, and on a bloated bureaucracy. We are no healthier than the citizens of comparable developed countries that spend half what we do and provide health care for everybody. In fact, by important measures such as life expectancy and infant mortality, the United States is far down the list.

If the wasted money could be redirected, the United States could include those now shut out of the system—without increasing the total outlay for health care and without restricting the availability of $100,000 bone-marrow transplants or $40,000 heart operations to those relatively few who need them.

"I can't imagine a system that's more dysfunctional than the one we have now—more expensive, not doing the job, with more waste," says Dr. Philip Caper, an internist and medical policy analyst at Dartmouth Medical School. Although the total amount of waste in our health care system is difficult to estimate, researchers have now examined many of the system's components, with consistent results. For a wide range of clinical procedures, on average, roughly 20 percent of the money we now spend could be saved with no loss in the quality of care. By restructuring the system, we could also save almost half of the huge amount we now spend on administrative costs. A more efficient system would also make it much easier to detect health care fraud—a problem that the U.S. General Accounting Office has estimated to cost tens of billions of dollars a year.

While these facts are well known to students of the health care system, they have been remarkably absent from the debate that is developing over health care in this election year. Politicians and lobbyists for health care providers have presented the public with a daunting choice: If we want to provide every American with access to health care, they say, we'll either have to pay much more into the system or have to accept lower-quality medical services.

However, such scenarios assume that the current price structure for medical care, and the current patterns of treatment and hospitalization, will remain fixed. They need not, and they should not. Our health care system is so inherently wasteful and inefficient that a complete overhaul is an option worth contemplating. It may, in fact, be the only option that makes sense.

The waste in the system comes from many sources. We receive a great deal of care that we do not need at all. The care we do need is delivered inefficiently. And the futile effort to control a runaway system has created a huge bureaucracy that by itself sucks up more than $100 billion a year.

THIRTY YEARS OF INCREASES

By now, it's hardly news that health costs have spiraled out of control. Health care now consumes about 16 percent of state and local tax revenues. In the years since 1986, private businesses have spent about as much on health care as they earned in after-tax profits. For many small businesses, insurance has become unaffordable; three out of four concerns employing 10 or fewer people simply do not provide health benefits. At any given time, roughly 35 million Americans—most of them employees of small businesses or their dependents—have no health coverage at all.

Over the last 10 years, government and private business, appalled to see health care absorbing an ever-growing portion of their revenues, have tried to get a grip on its costs in various ways. But costs have risen as fast as ever. "As quickly as payers patch the system up, the providers find the spaces between the patches," says Maryann O'Sullivan, director of Health Access, a California consumer coalition.

Our health care system does not just allow prices to rise—it practically demands that they do. Although some recent reforms have had a modest effect, the system has traditionally allowed doctors to order whatever procedures they want and has paid both doctors and hospitals whatever they think they should get.

In both respects, the American system stands alone in the developed world. Though the particulars of their systems differ, Canada, Japan, and the Western European countries all have adopted universal, standard payment schedules set by direct negotiation

---

"As quickly as payers patch the system up, the providers find the spaces between the patches."

---

with doctors and hospitals. In addition, most have set an overall ceiling on national medical expenditures. As a result, not a single developed country other than the United States devotes more than 10 percent of its gross national product to health care. The United States broke that barrier in 1985; in 1992, the nation is expected to spend 14 percent of the GNP on health.

It was not always so. In 1960, the United States spent a modest 5.3 percent of its GNP on health care, about the same as other industrialized nations like Canada or Germany did at the time. What changed everything was the advent in 1965 of Medicare, which ultimately had implications far beyond the over-65 population it served.

Before Medicare, private insurance companies covered the population less extensively than they do today. Insurers left treatment completely to the doctor's discretion and provided reimbursement for any test or treatment a physician ordered. But because a large percentage of people had only hospital coverage and no insurance to cover doctors' bills, physicians tended to keep fees at affordable levels.

In 1965, Congress enacted Medicare, the vast government-financed program of social health insurance for the elderly, along with the less extensive Medicaid program, in which the federal government shares costs with the states. In order to overcome the powerful, sustained opposition of doctors and hospitals to what they called "socialized medicine," Congress made a fateful—and, in retrospect, very expensive—decision. Under Medicare, all doctors were paid on the basis of their "usual and customary" fees for a given service (the system that Blue Shield was already using).

This approach, which allowed each individual physician to name his or her own price, soon became universal throughout the insurance industry. So, as more and more employers began offering major-medical plans that covered doctors' bills, they bought into a system with no effective constraints on costs. Predictably, doctors' fees began a rapid upward climb.

Hospitals profited as well. Under Blue Cross, which had dominated hospital insurance, hospitals were paid only a daily room charge, plus additional fees for various services, tests, and supplies. Under Medicare, however, the hospitals were not only able to collect their actual charges; for the first time, they were allowed to build the cost of capital improvements into their rates. Hospitals, which had been receiving federal subsidies for growth since the late 1940s, now got another incentive to expand.

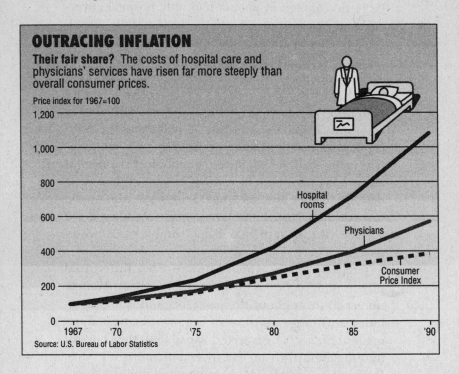

OUTRACING INFLATION

Their fair share? The costs of hospital care and physicians' services have risen far more steeply than overall consumer prices.

Price index for 1967=100

Hospital rooms

Physicians

Consumer Price Index

Source: U.S. Bureau of Labor Statistics

After Medicare, U.S. health care expenditures turned more sharply upward. For a time—perhaps a decade or more—no one seemed to notice or care.

But over the past 10 years or so, as costs have become truly staggering, the system has begun to change. Medicare has set limits on physicians' fees for several years, and private insurance companies have begun reviewing many of the procedures that doctors perform before they will pay for them. Medicaid budgets have been steadily cut back, to the point where many states now pay doctors and hospitals less than the cost of delivering care.

Experience has shown, however, that attempts to manage the health care system a piece at a time are likely to fail. Physicians and hospitals can charge their privately insured patients more to make up for Medicare's fee restrictions. And doctors and patients alike have resisted efforts by insurance companies to determine what is appropriate and necessary treatment, having grown used to a system that has provided as much medical care—to the insured population, that is—as anybody wants.

NO SENSE OF LIMITS

Having operated for years under a system that sets virtually no limit on what can be done or what can be charged, both doctors and patients have been seduced by the idea that, when it comes to treating sickness, it's necessary to do "everything."

"We want more. We want more time with the doctor. We want more procedures. We want more pills," says Randall Bovbjerg, a health policy analyst at the Urban Institute in Washington, D.C. "We can't sit and watch the course of a cold; we go and buy tons of things we aren't even certain will make it better."

"Imagine if we sold auto-purchase insurance and said, go buy whatever car you want, and we'll pay 80 percent of it," says James C. Robinson, a health care economist at the University of California, Berkeley. Under those conditions, a lot of people would go buy a Mercedes.

Much of the time, physicians will order more tests and procedures out of a genuine desire to do whatever they can for their patients. "Doctors look at one patient at a time and think, 'If I've done one thing, what else can I try?'," says Ann Lennarson Greer, a medical sociologist at the University of Wisconsin. "They're not inclined to think about overall costs." Several studies, in fact, have asked doctors if they knew the costs of hospital tests and services they routinely ordered, and the studies found many had only a vague idea at best.

But while extra tests and treatments drive up the cost of medical care, they may do so with no real benefit to the patient. New diagnostic technologies, in particular, are especially likely to be overused; unlike surgery or invasive procedures, they "don't require the clinician to take any real risk," Greer says. Thus, the use of computerized tomography (CT) and magnetic resonance imaging (MRI) scans, two expensive and relatively new imaging technologies, has grown explosively in recent years. Yet no one has clearly defined when they are useful and when they are a waste of time and money.

"The original CT scanner proved to be an absolute revolution in the treatment of patients with head injury," says Dr. Mark Chassin, a physician who is senior vice-president of Value Health Sciences, a private firm that analyzes the use of health care services. "We produced hundreds of these things and they got out in the community. They were used for people with head trauma—terrific—but they also were used for people with headaches, dizziness, and all sorts of other vague symptoms." Diagnostic imaging, says Dr. Chassin, is a prime example of how "we continue to invest in technology in an absolutely irrational way."

THE LAW OF INDUCED DEMAND

Medical care is unlike services delivered by other professionals. When clients hire an architect or a lawyer, they generally know what they need and roughly how much it's going to cost. But in medicine, physicians make virtually all the decisions that determine the cost of care. The patient, ill and uninformed, is neither in a position to do comparison shopping, nor motivated to weigh the costs, so long as insurance is paying the bill.

The more services doctors perform, the more they get paid, a situation that is tailor-made for cost escalation. "It's the easiest thing in the world to increase the volume [of things a doctor does]," says Dr. Philip Caper, the Dartmouth internist. "Just do a few more tests. There's always a rationale. Schedule three doctor visits instead of two and reduce the time you spend on each visit."

Something like this may have happened in the mid-1980s, when Medicare abruptly froze physicians' fees. In 1986, in the midst of the freeze, doctors managed to collect 15 percent more in Medicare fees than

11

they had the year before. The creation of medical "need" by those who then profit from it is called *induced demand*, and it's rampant. Most obvious is the problem of self-referral, in which physicians will send patients for treatment to facilities in which they have a financial interest.

In Florida, where at least 40 percent of the physicians have such investments, a study by professors at Florida State University found that physician-owned laboratories performed twice as many tests per patient as independent labs. Similarly, in a University of Arizona study of private health insurance claims for more than 65,000 patients, researchers found that doctors who had diagnostic imaging equipment in their offices ordered four times more imaging exams than doctors who referred patients elsewhere for the tests.

Occasionally, self-referral can turn into actual fraud. A recent General Accounting Office report, which estimated that fraud may account for as much as 10 percent of all health care costs, cited several examples in which self-referral had been abused. In one California case, owners of mobile medical laboratories allegedly gave kickbacks for referrals to physicians who sometimes used phony diagnoses to justify the tests. The case, still under investigation, involves an estimated $1 billion in fraudulent billings.

In other cases, however, physicians may increase the demand for their services without even being aware of it. When it comes to American medical care, supply seems to create demand almost automatically. Actuarial studies have shown that in areas with the greatest supply of physicians, people simply go to the doctor more often. If more physicians create more demand for medical care, we can look forward to a flood of it in the near future. The per capita supply of practicing physicians is expected to increase 22 percent between now and the year 2000.

The phenomenon of induced demand applies to hospitals, too. Dr. John Wennberg, a professor of family and community medicine at Dartmouth Medical School, was curious as to why people in Boston went to the hospital more frequently than people in New Haven, Connecticut. When he studied the problem, he found a simple answer: Boston has more hospital beds to be filled — one-third more than New Haven on a per capita basis.

Surprisingly, Dr. Wennberg found that physicians in Boston and New Haven were completely unaware of the discrepancy. When he asked doctors in New Haven whether they felt their area was short of hospital beds, they said they did not. In fact, at any given time, about 85 percent of the hospital beds in New Haven were filled, precisely the same percentage as in Boston.

The likely explanation, according to Dr. Wennberg, is that physicians almost unconsciously will refer their patients to the hospital if space is available, stopping only when the local hospitals' capacity is nearly used up. If many beds are empty, doctors will be more likely to refer patients with borderline conditions, such as gastroenteritis or acute low-back pain, for which hospitalization is optional but not imperative. By doing so, of course, they drive up the cost of care.

AN UNNECESSARY BURDEN

With so many incentives to overtreat patients, it seems inevitable that a sizable fraction of American medical care must be simply unnecessary, if not downright harmful. But how large a fraction? In the late 1970s and early 1980s, researchers at the Rand Corporation, a think tank in Santa Monica, California, began to find out.

Using an elaborate process for developing a consensus among nationally recognized medical experts, the Rand team came up with an agreed-upon list of "indications" for various procedures. They then checked the actual medical records of thousands of patients who had received the procedures, to see whether they had been treated appropriately. The definition of "appropriate" care was starkly simple: Based on the patient's condition and expert opinion, the likely benefit of the procedure must have been greater than the risk involved in doing it.

Even with their elaborate analysis, the Rand researchers were not able to tell in every case whether a given procedure had been appropriate or not. They divided their cases into three groups: Those for which the procedure had been "appropriate," for which it was "inappropriate," and for which its use was "equivocal," the largest group. Despite this degree of uncertainty, however, Rand found clear evidence of inappropriate overtreatment. Among the results:

- Of 1,300 elderly patients who had an operation to remove atherosclerotic plaque from the carotid artery, 32 percent, or nearly one-third, did not need it.

- Of 386 heart bypass operations, 14 percent were done unnecessarily.
- Of 1,677 patients who had coronary angiography (an X-ray examination of blood flow in the arteries nourishing the heart), 17 percent didn't need it.

So striking were the results that Rand's methods for determining appropriateness have since been put to commercial use. Value Health Sciences, which now employs some of the original Rand researchers, has extended the methodology to several dozen high-volume medical procedures. A number of major insurance companies and health maintenance organizations now use this program to flag unnecessary procedures.

Value Health's results confirm the original Rand findings. Its review system has found very high rates of unnecessary usage for certain procedures: hysterectomy, 27 percent unnecessary; surgery for carpal tunnel syndrome, an uncomfortable wrist ailment, 17 percent; tonsillectomy, 16 percent; laminectomy, a type of back surgery, 14 percent. Similar results have come out of studies done by other investigators, who have examined procedures from preoperative laboratory screening (60 percent unnecessary) to cesarean section (50 percent unnecessary) to upper gastrointestinal X-ray studies (30 percent unnecessary).

THE UNCERTAINTY PRINCIPLE

Physicians can inadvertently contribute to the cost of health care even when they have only their patients' best interest in mind. Lay people tend to think of medical care as a straightforward proposition: For Disease A, prescribe Treatment B. But in real life, to practice medicine is to be afloat in a "sea of uncertainty," says Dartmouth's John Wennberg.

Every symptom can be investigated by a huge array of tests, and for many diseases, physicians have a wide range of treatment choices. And doctors often base their choices as much on folklore and intuition as on science. "Doctors really hate risks," says Ann Lennarson Greer, the Wisconsin sociologist. "They have certain procedures that seem to work for them, and they'd prefer to keep doing them, especially in areas where there's a lot of uncertainty."

This innate conservatism is reinforced by the isolation in which most doctors practice, says Greer, who has spent more than a decade studying why doctors and hospitals behave as they do. A physician can spend his or her entire career within a single referral network, based at a single hospital. Local colleagues, Greer has found, are the principal influence on a physician's decisions about how to diagnose and treat diseases or whether or not to adopt new technology. But they may not be the most reliable resource.

A phenomenon called "small area variation," which was discovered by Dr. Wennberg early in his career, is a striking demonstration of just how unscientific medical practice really is. In the late 1960s, he had moved to Vermont to work as a health administrator and educator. Once there, he soon stumbled across a curious geographic pattern to a common operation, tonsillectomy.

"In Stowe, the probability of having a tonsillectomy by age 15 was about 70 percent," Dr. Wennberg recalls. "If you lived in Waterbury, over the hill from Stowe, it was about 10 percent." Indeed, there turned out to be a 13-fold difference in the local rates of tonsillectomy between the most and the least surgery-happy Vermont communities he studied.

Medical uncertainty and the isolation of doctors largely explain those bizarre disparities. Dr. Wennberg discovered that doctors in Stowe, who talked mostly to each other, believed that if you did not remove the tonsils early, they would become chronically infected and cause no end of trouble. Doctors in Waterbury, who did not talk to the doctors in Stowe, held the opposite (and, as it turned out, correct) viewpoint: If left alone, most kids with frequent sore throats would eventually outgrow them.

This phenomenon turned out to be true of a lot more than tonsillectomies. In Portland, Maine, Dr. Wennberg found, 50 percent of men had prostate surgery by the age of 85; in Bangor, just 10 percent did. The rate of heart surgery was twice as high in Des Moines as it was in nearby Iowa City. Subsequent studies by a number of researchers working throughout the country have shown that the use of all kinds of medical procedures varies dramatically from region to region. In fact, Dr. Wennberg has found

17

that the only procedures that *do not* show such variations are those few for which there is basically only
one accepted treatment, such as hospitalization for
heart attack or stroke.

INEFFICIENCY STUDIES

The waste in the system goes far beyond the provision of unnecessary care. Even when medical treatments are necessary, they are frequently done with
no regard for efficiency.

Milliman and Robertson, a Seattle-based consulting
firm, advises hospitals and other health care organizations on ways to cut costs without compromising
the quality of care. The firm's actuaries and physicians have examined thousands of individual medical
records to develop guidelines on how long patients
should stay in the hospital for such common conditions as childbirth or appendectomy, provided they
are in generally good health and have no complications. Applying those guidelines to actual current
records from a dozen urban areas across the country,
the firm's actuaries concluded that 53 percent of all
hospital days were unnecessary, including all the days
spent in the hospital by the 24 percent of patients
who did not need to be there in the first place.

As a private, commercial firm, Milliman and
Robertson is in business to identify overuse for its
clients, so it might have a bias in favor of finding
what it is paid to find. However, other studies by academic researchers have also found high rates of inappropriate hospitalization. A recent Rand Corporation
review of published studies, most of which used data

from the early and middle 1980s, estimated that 15 to 30 percent of hospital use was unnecessary.

The current rates of unnecessary hospitalization are difficult to estimate, since the system is in flux. The overall number of hospital days per thousand Americans—a standard measure of hospital utilization—has dropped over the last decade, largely in response to efforts by Medicare, health maintenance organizations, and private insurers to contain costs. But there are still large regional variations in hospital use, suggesting that waste still exists in the system.

Past experience shows it's possible to lower the number of days people spend in hospitals, with no ill effects. In 1984, Medicare created financial incentives for hospitals to discharge patients as soon as possible and not to admit them at all unless strictly necessary. The incentives worked; in two years, the average number of in-patient days per Medicare recipient fell 22 percent.

That sharp decline apparently had no real impact on the health of the patients involved, according to several statistics. The rate at which discharged patients need to be readmitted to the hospital shortly after leaving—an important index of low-quality care—has actually gone down for Medicare patients since 1984. Some care that used to be provided in the hospital can now be provided at home, at much lower cost.

A MEDICAL 'ARMS RACE'

Despite the efforts over the past decade to keep the costs of hospitalization down by limiting hospital admissions, length of stay, and in-patient costs, our national hospital bill continues to rise. In 1990, hospitals soaked up 38 percent of national health expenditures (twice as much as doctors) and collectively earned a profit of $7 billion. Hospital administrators have proven how nimble health care providers can be in getting around virtually any effort to rein them in.

For many years, hospitals expanded at a rate well beyond the national need, and with the government's help. During the 1950s and into the 1960s, the federal government provided subsidies to build new hospitals. A decade later, Medicare allowed hospitals to pay for their capital improvements by charging higher fees. The result was a spate of hospital-building that had little relationship to perceivable community needs. New facilities and new wings were built, so beds needed to be filled, and the law of induced demand kept them occupied, imposing a high cost on the health care system and providing a high profit for the hospitals themselves.

When Medicare started to crack down on costs in 1984 by paying hospitals a fixed fee to take care of each patient, based on his or her diagnosis, the hospitals reacted swiftly. Fewer Medicare patients were admitted, and those that were admitted stayed in the hospital for a shorter time. But the hospitals compensated by boosting their outpatient, psychiatric, and rehabilitation services, for which Medicare had set no cost limits. Although charges for hospitalization dropped, the costs for those other services ate up the savings, and more.

Hospitals also stepped up their efforts to attract privately insured patients to make up for the money they were losing on Medicare and Medicaid. Having built the capacity for many more beds than the nation needs, hospitals now tried to fill them—and with patients who had generous insurance policies and needed many medical services. "Hospitals make money by delivering services," explains William Erwin, spokesman for the American Hospital Association. "If you don't need much done to you, the hospital isn't going to make money on you."

Attracting patients to a hospital is not the same as attracting customers to a new restaurant or hardware store. Consumers decide on their own when and where they want to eat out or buy some drill bits. When they are sick, their doctors decide when and where to hospitalize them. So hospitals must market

---

"Hospitals make money by delivering services. If you don't need much done to you, the hospital isn't going to make money on you."

---

on two fronts: They must appeal directly to privately insured patients, and they must keep their admitting doctors happy.

To induce physicians to admit patients, hospitals resort to everything from first-year guaranteed incomes to subsidies for initial practice expenses. The effort pays off. In 1990, according to an annual survey by Jackson and Coker, an Atlanta physician-recruiting firm, the average doctor generated $513,000 in in-patient hospital revenue.

Another way to keep doctors happy is to provide them with state-of-the-art medical equipment. As a bonus, hospitals can then tout their up-to-date technology directly to consumers. Uwe Reinhardt, a Princeton University health economist, likes to paint the following scenario in his lectures:

"Imagine that you're a young couple in Chicago, stuck in a traffic jam in the Loop, and you see a billboard that says: 'Sacred Heart: The Cheapest Place in Chicago. Have Your Baby Here.' Then you see another billboard that says, 'Holy Mercy: The Only Place with a Glandular Schlumpulator. Have Your Baby Here.' Where are you going to go?"

Some regulatory efforts were made in the 1960s and 1970s to restrain hospitals from acquiring excessive amounts of expensive technology, with mixed success. Federal support for that effort was discontinued during the Reagan years. The rationale was that "unleashing competition" among hospitals would allow the free market to operate and help keep the cost of medicine down.

The irony is that, where hospitals are concerned, competition actually drives costs up. The hospitals gain no competitive advantage by controlling costs, since their customers—doctors and patients—are not the ones paying for their services anyway. Instead, hospitals compete only on the basis of perceived quality, and they end up vying to see which one can secure and promote the newest well-reimbursed technology, whether needed or not. Several hospitals in an area may have their own neonatal intensive care units, MRI machines, or cardiac care centers, when only one would serve the population equally well. In 1992, despite the recession, hospitals plan to increase spending on new equipment by 15 percent, according to a survey by Shearson Lehman Brothers.

To attract the well-insured population, hospitals also provide amenities that have nothing to do with actual health care but add to the bill, including cable TV, private rooms and baths, gourmet menus, and the like. Baylor University Medical Center in Houston spent $18 million on the Tom Landry Sports Medicine and Research Center, complete with 7,000-square-foot dressing rooms lined with oak lockers and a 10-lane pool with underwater computerized video cameras used to analyze its patrons' swimming strokes.

Hospitals have also become more and more consciously concerned with projecting an upscale image that they hope will bring in an affluent clientele. Entries in a recent contest held by the Academy of Health Services Marketing, an organization of hospital marketing executives, reveal the new focus. For instance, the Southern Regional Medical Center in suburban Atlanta got Rosalynn Carter, the former First Lady, to endorse its maternity service after her grandchild was born there; this was part of a successful campaign "to increase gross revenue . . . by marketing to a target market of insured, higher-income women, ages 25–49," according to the contest submission.

The trend is troubling because there is clear evidence that the total cost of health care rises in areas where many hospitals begin to compete for the same well-insured patients. Health economists James C. Robinson and Harold S. Luft of the University of California, Berkeley, examined data from 5,732 hospitals nationwide and found that costs per admission were 26 percent higher in hospitals that had more than nine competitors within a 15-mile radius. In a smaller-scale study of 747 hospitals, they found that those in competitive areas allowed patients to stay in the hospital longer after surgery—something that tends to please both patients and doctors, but at a high cost and with no clear medical benefit.

THE CARDIAC MONEY MACHINE

The treatment of heart and circulatory diseases, the leading causes of death in the nation, illustrates as well as anything the manner in which the current U.S. system promotes expensive, dubious care. People suffering from these diseases have benefited enormously from medical and surgical advances over the past two decades. Until the late 1960s, doctors could do little more than give them some nitroglycerin or digitalis in the hope of extending their lives moderately. Then came coronary bypass surgery, the first great advance, in which blood vessels taken from elsewhere in the body are used to bypass diseased coronary vessels and restore ample blood supply to the heart muscle. Next, in the 1980s, balloon angioplasty was developed, in which a balloon attached to a catheter is passed into the narrowed coronary vessel and inflated to crush the blockage against the wall of the coronary artery.

The last decade has also brought new drugs to dissolve blood clots, to correct irregular heartbeats, and to treat heart failure and high blood pressure; new imaging techniques; implantable electronic devices; and, as a last resort, new methods of heart transplantation.

All this, together with changes in diet and exercise habits, has had a dramatic effect. The death rate from heart disease in the United States has dropped by roughly half since 1950.

But the improvement has come at a very high cost. New technologies are expensive technologies, and the cardiac field is no exception. Coronary bypass surgery, for example, can easily run $30,000 or more for a single operation.

"It is just well paid by everybody; even Medicare pays handsomely for it," says Ann Greer, the Wisconsin medical sociologist. "The hospitals are crazy about bypass. Even if they're six blocks from a major heart center, they think they can't afford not to be in on it." The people who develop coronary problems predominantly are middle-aged men, who tend to be the best-insured people in our society. Uninsured patients, meanwhile, may miss out on these costly procedures. One national survey found they were 39 percent less likely than the insured to get coronary angiograms, which are X-rays to evaluate the heart's blood supply, and 29 percent less likely to have bypass surgery.

A GROWING PROFIT CENTER

Just how lucrative is the cardiovascular field was revealed in a 1990 report prepared by the Advisory Board Company, a Washington-based consulting firm, for its hospital clients. The report concludes that nearly one-quarter of all hospital revenues come from cardiology-related business, and of that, more than 80 percent comes from just four procedures: cardiac catheterization, angioplasty, bypass surgery, and heart-valve surgery. Not surprisingly, cardiovascular surgeons bring in the most annual revenue per inpatient admittance of any specialty. At $10,942 in 1989, it was at more than twice the average doctor's rate, according to a survey by Jackson and Coker, an Atlanta-based physician-recruiting firm.

The profit margins are as impressive as the revenues, according to the Advisory Board report: 70 percent for catheterization, 37 percent for angioplasty, and 40 percent for bypass, compared with overall hospital profit margins of less than 4 percent. To top it all off, the number of cardiac diagnostic and treatment procedures performed in the United States has been growing at an average annual rate of 12.7 percent.

The Advisory Board report uses a real, though unidentified, hospital to illustrate the profit potential. Wanting to increase its cardiology market share, the hospital invested $3 million in state-of-the-art equipment for catheterization and open-heart surgery. The improved equipment (and additional support staff) attracted 25 new cardiologists to the hospital, who brought in hundreds of new patients for catheterization, angioplasty, and bypass. Within two years, the extra business had repaid the entire up-front investment and was adding $1.8 million a year in profits to the hospital's bottom line.

This sort of return on investment has caused hospitals to look increasingly to cardiovascular care to fill their empty beds. In 1980, according to the Advisory

Board report, there were 382,000 cardiac catheterizations performed in the U.S. and 340,000 treatment procedures, including bypass, angioplasty, valve surgery, and pacemaker implantations. By 1988, the volume of catheterizations had grown to 965,000 and the volume of the other procedures to 930,000.

Were all those procedures really necessary?

DOCTORS' DILEMMAS

The treatment of heart disease is a classic example of the way in which medical uncertainty produces variable, unnecessary care. Treatments for heart disease are advancing so rapidly that there is often little consensus on what to do or when to do it. What symptoms require a coronary angiography exam? Should a person with mildly uncomfortable angina and blockages in one or two vessels stick with drug treatment or undergo angioplasty? If angioplasty has failed once, should it be repeated or should the patient get a bypass operation?

Medical journals are filled with debates on these questions. In the meantime, physicians must make daily treatment decisions with little guidance on which course is preferable, but knowing that they will be financially rewarded for ordering the maximum intervention.

Writing in the *Journal of the American Medical Association*, Dr. Thomas N. James of the University of Texas, Galveston, put it this way: "The same physician who decides whether a diagnostic or therapeutic procedure is to be done is too often also the one who does the procedure, interprets the findings (and

27

decides whether additional procedures are indicated), and is paid for each step of the way. This is not to say that such physicians are unskillful or that their decisions are necessarily made on the basis of personal gain, but the temptation is inescapably there."

Under those circumstances, it would be surprising if unnecessary procedures were not being done. The evidence is that they are. Consider the following:

- A study of pacemaker implantations in Philadelphia hospitals found that 20 percent were unnecessary and another 36 percent were problematic.

- A San Diego team found that, among patients who had been hospitalized with mild heart attacks, 40 percent of those who got angiograms did not need them. In addition to running up a bill ranging from $2,000 to $3,500, the procedure put patients at a slight risk of complications.

- A team from Brigham and Women's Hospital in Boston examined the need for bypass surgery among 88 patients for whom it had been recommended. They advised against surgery for 74 of the 88. Among those 74, 60 accepted the second opinion and did not have the operation. Over a follow-up period of more than two years, there were only two subsequent heart attacks, neither of them fatal, among this group—an outcome comparable to that of people who receive angioplasty or coronary bypass surgery.

RISKY MEDICINE

Despite findings like these, competitive and financial pressures conspire to encourage hospitals to build even more cardiac care units. Consider the case of Manchester, New Hampshire. Until 1985, Manchester residents who needed open-heart surgery had to travel to Boston or to Hanover, New Hampshire, to get it. That year, a Manchester hospital, Catholic Hospital Medical Center, opened the first local open-heart surgery service. Within one year, the rate of heart surgery among residents of Manchester more than doubled.

What could explain the immediate jump in volume? An analysis by the Codman Research Group, a private health care consulting firm, found that before the local program started, 90 percent of the bypasses done on Manchester residents involved the transplantation of three or more arteries—a sign of serious and extensive disease. By 1988, however, over half the operations were single or double bypasses.

"They were clearly operating on less severely ill patients," says Dr. Philip Caper, Codman's chairman and a professor at Dartmouth Medical School. "The hooker is, nobody really knows whether they were better off. Some doctors think most single bypasses should almost never be done, because the risk is greater than the benefit."

While coronary bypass can be lifesaving, it is an extremely traumatic procedure involving stopping and cooling the heart, hooking the patient up to a heart-lung machine, then restarting the heart. Handling an operation of this complexity requires a skilled and coordinated surgical team. That is why studies have repeatedly demonstrated that hospitals performing fewer than 150 open-heart procedures a year have higher death rates than those that perform more. In addition to driving up health care costs, hospitals joining the cardiac gold rush may actually be putting their patients at serious risk.

That was the case in Phoenix in 1985, when the state of Arizona, in the spirit of deregulation, decided to abdicate its authority to control the introduction of new open-heart surgery programs. At that time, four Phoenix hospitals provided open-heart surgery. Almost immediately, seven more began programs. A computer-aided study of Medicare records performed by the Phoenix *Gazette* and the University of Arizona found that in the first year of deregulation the local death rate from heart surgery increased by 35 percent. The average cost of the procedure, meanwhile, rose 50 percent.

MORE SPECIALISTS, HIGHER COSTS

Just as American hospitals lead the world in high-priced technology, American physicians are heavy purveyors of expensive treatments and diagnostic tests, and they reap great personal rewards for using them. Doctors in the United States earn much higher incomes relative to their fellow citizens than do doctors in other countries. According to figures from the Organization for Economic Cooperation and Devel-

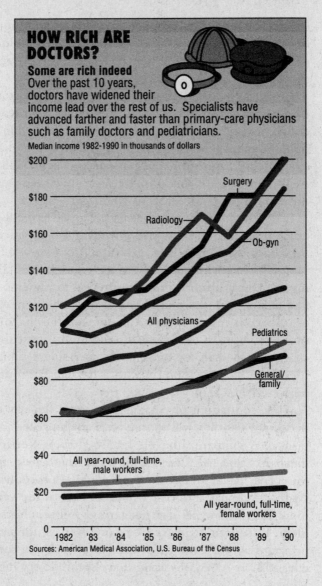

HOW RICH ARE DOCTORS?

Some are rich indeed
Over the past 10 years, doctors have widened their income lead over the rest of us. Specialists have advanced farther and faster than primary-care physicians such as family doctors and pediatricians.

Median income 1982-1990 in thousands of dollars

Surgery
Radiology
Ob-gyn
All physicians
Pediatrics
General/family

All year-round, full-time, male workers
All year-round, full-time, female workers

1982 '83 '84 '85 '86 '87 '88 '89 '90

Sources: American Medical Association, U.S. Bureau of the Census

opment, in 1987 U.S. doctors earned 5.4 times more than the average worker. In Germany, the multiple was 4.2; in Canada, 3.7; and in France, Japan, and the United Kingdom, 2.4.

Historically, the highest fees have gone to doctors who perform concrete procedures such as surgery, endoscopy, or diagnostic imaging. So-called evaluation and management services, in which doctors may examine and question the patient and prescribe a treatment, but do not actually do a specific procedure, have not paid nearly as well.

In 1990, for instance, internists charged a median of $110 for a comprehensive office visit for a patient they had not seen before, according to a survey by *Medical Economics* magazine. Such a visit involves taking a medical history, doing a physical examination, and talking with the patient about his or her current condition. It can take up 45 minutes of the doctor's time. By contrast, the same survey found internists charged a median fee of $126 for spending 10 minutes to examine the bowel with a flexible fiberoptic device called a sigmoidoscope.

While individual physicians have great leeway in deciding what they will charge for a given procedure, insurance companies have established computerized databanks that help them determine whether or not the fee is "usual and customary" for that procedure. By this standard, a doctor whose fees are at the very top of the local scale may not receive full reimbursement. But there is no "track record" of cost for new procedures. With the help of medical specialty societies and the AMA, physicians have secured very high rates of reimbursement for new treatments.

"When something is in development, it's new, it's experimental, only a few physicians use it, there's some risk involved, and the price gets set accordingly," explains Joel Cantor, a program officer at the Robert Wood Johnson Foundation. "Then the technology diffuses and gets easier to use. More physicians get good at it. But the price never goes down."

The classic example is the extraction of cataracts and implantation of artificial lenses in the eye. This undeniably useful technology was introduced in the early 1980s and became a standard procedure by the end of the decade. During that time, however, many ophthalmologists became wealthy by charging $2,000 or more for a cataract extraction that could be done in about an hour.

Primary-care physicians, such as general internists, family practitioners, and pediatricians, do few such procedures; instead, they spend their days in office visits, which have long-established, and thus lower, "usual and customary" fee profiles. As a result, their incomes are much lower than those of specialists. In 1990, the median income for general family practitioners was $93,000, and for pediatricians, $100,000, according to the American Medical Association's annual survey. Median income for surgeons and radiologists, on the other hand, was $200,000. Senior specialists can earn much, much more. Cardiovascular surgeons in group practice averaged about $500,000 in 1990, according to a study by the Medical Group Management Association.

Medical students, who must pick a residency program in their senior year, are painfully aware of these economic distinctions. In addition, they are trained in an academic environment that has long rewarded specialists with prestige and research grants. Young physicians, who leave medical school with a huge debt load, are increasingly turning to specialization. Overall, about one-third of U.S. physicians are in primary care. But among 1987 medical school graduates who have now completed their internships and residencies, only one-fourth have gone into primary care, according to data from the Association of American Medical Colleges.

A fed-up Ohio family doctor, responding to a survey by his professional society, the American Academy of Family Physicians, summarized his feelings this way: "Why bother with 60- to 70-hour work weeks, constant phone calls, all-night emergency room visits, poor reimbursements, demanding patients, the need for instant, exact decisions . . . concerning a million possible diseases, when you can 'specialize' in one organ, get paid $500 for a 15-minute procedure, only need to know a dozen drugs and side effects, and work part-time?"

Do we really need our luxurious quantities of cardiologists, dermatologists, neurosurgeons, and urologists? Other countries get along fine with about a 50–50 ratio between primary-care doctors and specialists. The evidence is that we could, too.

A team from the New England Medical Center recently looked at patients who got their usual care from primary-care physicians (internists or family doctors) or from specialists (cardiologists and endocrinologists). The groups were not identical; the specialists tended to have older patients with more medical problems. But even after that difference was factored in, the specialists ran up higher bills, on average, than the primary-care doctors. They put more patients in the hospital, prescribed more drugs, and performed more tests. An analysis still in progress appears to show that the two groups of patients had similar health outcomes.

The medical profession itself acknowledges the imbalance. The principal professional journal for internists, the *Annals of Internal Medicine*, said in a 1991 editorial: "Given the number of subspecialists already in practice, there are not enough highly specialized cases to go around. . . . We cannot continue to practice this way when cost containment is the dominant health policy issue of our times."

"Given the number of subspecialists already in practice, there are not enough highly specialized cases to go around. . . . We cannot continue to practice this way when cost containment is the dominant health policy issue of our times."

This year, Medicare began an effort to even out the economic imbalance between primary-care and specialty physicians. The new program, known as the Resource-Based Relative Value Scale (RBRVS), is essentially a standard national fee schedule, adjusted for geographic variations in the cost of practice. It increases the reimbursement for evaluation and management services and greatly reduces the reimburse-

Malpractice: A Straw Man

One factor commonly supposed to contribute to the high U.S. health care tab is malpractice. Ask physicians to explain why the cost of health care goes up continually, and they are likely to complain that the U.S. malpractice system encourages unnecessary "defensive" medical care.

The public seems to have bought this argument. In a recent survey, *Consumer Reports* subscribers guessed that malpractice tied with hospital costs as the biggest factor driving the cost of health care. But is malpractice such a villain?

It's true that malpractice costs are higher in the United States than in other countries. And in the mid-1980s, malpractice claims—and, accordingly, insurance premiums—did take a sharp upward swing. There was much talk then of a malpractice "crisis." But that crisis now seems to have abated, as have previous ones. Malpractice is a cyclical phenomenon; periodically, the incidence of claims rises, then falls back.

At the moment, malpractice claims are in a downward swing. The rate of claims has declined steadily since the peak of the last "crisis" in 1985. So have

malpractice insurance premiums. In 1990, according
to *Medical Economics* magazine's annual survey of
physicians, doctors' malpractice premiums on average consumed only 3.7 percent of their practice
receipts (though the percentage may be double that
for high-risk, and high-paid, specialties, such as
obstetrics, surgery, and anesthesiology). The U.S.
Department of Health and Human Services puts the
total cost of malpractice at less than 1 percent of total
health outlays.

But then, no one argues that the direct cost of malpractice insurance is the main factor driving up the
cost of care. Instead, it is assumed that physicians,
fearing malpractice suits, are forced to practice
"defensive medicine" just to protect themselves in the
event of a lawsuit.

Defensive medicine undoubtedly exists, and doctors themselves feel that the threat of malpractice
forces them to do more tests than are truly necessary.
But quantifying the cost of defensive medicine is a
slippery matter. The American Medical Association
made a stab at it in the 1980s and decided that the
total cost of medical malpractice, including premiums

and defensive medicine, was about 17 percent of physicians' earnings.

However, the AMA estimate was based on physicians' own reports of what they considered defensive practices, such as doing more diagnostic tests, sticking with the safest possible treatments, telling patients more about treatment risks, and keeping more complete records. As that list suggests, one problem with defining defensive medicine, let alone measuring it, is that it is difficult to distinguish from care delivered for other reasons. Is a doctor doing an unnecessary test out of fear of a lawsuit, or because the medical culture values doing "everything," or simply to reassure an anxious patient? Did an obstetrician perform an unnecessary cesarean for legal protection, for scheduling convenience, or to earn a higher fee?

"You mostly get anecdotes when you're talking about defensive medicine," says Randall Bovbjerg of the Urban Institute in Washington, D.C., who has worked on several malpractice studies. That's not to say there is no malpractice crisis, however: "The greatest single problem about malpractice is that there's a lot more of it out there than anyone is dealing with," says Bovbjerg. "Patients are getting avoidable injuries, and no one is stopping it."

Documentation for Bovbjerg's claim comes from a study conducted by Harvard University researchers for the state of New York. The researchers reviewed

a random sample of New York hospital records in 1984 and found that 3.7 percent of patients suffered "adverse events," slightly more than one-quarter of which could be attributed to actual negligence. Of those who suffered negligent injuries, only about one-eighth ever filed malpractice claims, and only about one-sixteenth ever recovered any damages. Conversely, the study found many cases in which patients filed malpractice suits with no clear evidence of negligence.

Costs aside, the current malpractice system is at best only an imprecise means of controlling the quality of medical care.

ment for procedures. Physicians, however, may find a way around this constraint, as they have around others. For one thing, doctors can always simply raise their fees for privately insured, non-Medicare patients, although some private insurance companies may eventually adopt a version of the RBRVS fee schedule.

Since the mid-1980s, doctors have also manipulated the reimbursement system by "unbundling" services— that is, by charging for two or more separate procedures instead of one. For instance, instead of billing $1,200 for a hysterectomy, a doctor can collect $7,000 by billing separately for various components of the operation. Commercial services conduct seminars to teach doctors how to maximize reimbursement in this way. But unbundling can cross the line into outright, prosecutable fraud, according to the General Accounting Office's report on health care fraud.

SUPPLIER-SIDE ECONOMICS

Just as the providers of care have profited hugely over the years, so have those who supply the providers: the pharmaceutical companies and the makers of medical equipment and devices. They can charge top prices for their products, secure in the knowledge that the system will reimburse them. The pharmaceutical industry has been one of the nation's most profitable industrial sectors; it operates with an average profit margin of 15 percent and has given an average annual return to investors of 25 percent over the last decade.

Companies that latch on to new medical technologies can also earn huge profits. In spite of the current hand-wringing over health care reform, as a group health care stocks increased in value by fully 50 percent in 1991. The Health Industry Manufacturers Association, a medical-equipment trade group, projects a 7.4-percent annual growth rate for health technology throughout the 1990s, provided that "negative scenarios" such as health care reform do not interfere. "A lot of people in health care are making a lot of money," says Stephen Zuckerman, a senior research associate at the Urban Institute in Washington, D.C. "They're not unhappy with the current system."

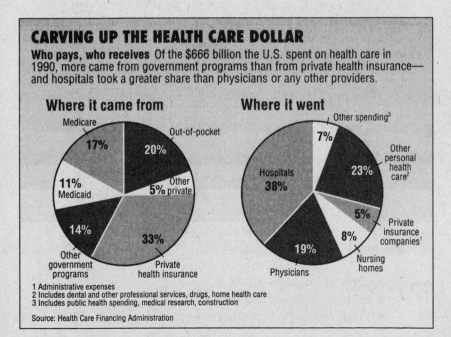

CARVING UP THE HEALTH CARE DOLLAR

Who pays, who receives Of the $666 billion the U.S. spent on health care in 1990, more came from government programs than from private health insurance— and hospitals took a greater share than physicians or any other providers.

Where it came from

- Medicare 17%
- Out-of-pocket 20%
- Other private 5%
- Medicaid 11%
- Other government programs 14%
- Private health insurance 33%

Where it went

- Other spending[3] 7%
- Other personal health care[2] 23%
- Private insurance companies[1] 5%
- Nursing homes 8%
- Physicians 19%
- Hospitals 38%

1 Administrative expenses
2 Includes dental and other professional services, drugs, home health care
3 Includes public health spending, medical research, construction

Source: Health Care Financing Administration

Curiously, the debate over health care costs tends to assume that the cost of drugs and medical technology is immutably fixed. But international comparisons demonstrate that this need not be so. In Japan, for example, the national fee schedule pays $177 for a magnetic resonance imaging (MRI) exam, compared with an average charge of about $1,000 in the United States. Pharmaceutical prices, which vary widely from country to country, are also significantly higher here than they are anywhere else.

NOTHING FOR SOMETHING

As costly as it is, our health care system might be worth its price if it somehow ended up making us healthier than people in other countries. But it does not.

Of the 24 industrialized nations making up the Organization for Economic Cooperation and Development (OECD), the United States spends more than twice as much on health per capita as is the average and devotes a far greater percentage of its gross national product to health care than any other country. Yet the other OECD countries—with the exception of Turkey and Greece, by far the poorest of the group—have roughly as many doctors and hospitals per capita as we do.

As for health status, of the 24 OECD countries, the United States ranks:

- 21st in infant mortality
- 17th in male life expectancy
- 16th in female life expectancy.

Dr. Barbara Starfield of the Johns Hopkins School of Public Health compared the United States with nine industrialized European nations in three areas: the availability of high-quality primary care, public

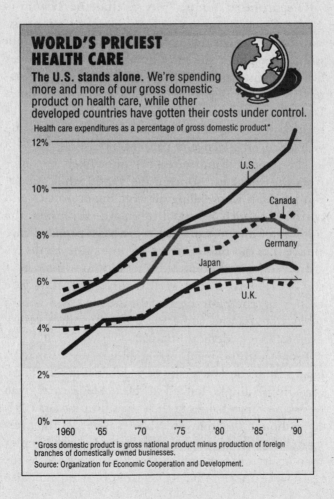

WORLD'S PRICIEST HEALTH CARE

The U.S. stands alone. We're spending more and more of our gross domestic product on health care, while other developed countries have gotten their costs under control.

Health care expenditures as a percentage of gross domestic product*

*Gross domestic product is gross national product minus production of foreign branches of domestically owned businesses.

Source: Organization for Economic Cooperation and Development.

health indicators such as infant mortality and life expectancy, and overall public satisfaction with the value of health care. In all three areas, the United States ranked at or near the bottom.

The problem, simply put, is that the system is geared to providing the services that can'earn physicians and hospitals the most money, not the ones that will do the public the most good. The United States has four times as many $1.5-million magnetic resonance imaging devices per capita as Germany does. But at the same time, the U.S. system shortchanges many types of basic, low-tech care that have, over the years, proven effective at preventing disease.

The poor and uninsured are most likely to suffer from the imbalance. During the 1980s, while American hospitals were falling all over themselves to add costly, high-tech neonatal intensive-care units, the number of mothers unable to get basic prenatal care climbed, as did the incidence of premature births.

In most states, Medicaid now pays nowhere near the actual cost of delivering care; hospitals lose money on their Medicaid admissions. As a result, many doctors and some for-profit hospitals refuse even to accept Medicaid patients.

People with no insurance at all fare even worse. A group from the University of California at San Francisco, for example, looked at the hospital care given to sick newborn babies in the state's hospitals in 1987. Even though the uninsured babies were, on the average, the sickest group, they left the hospital sooner than insured babies and received fewer services while they were there. The Rand Corporation has also shown that when California cut back on Medicaid coverage a decade ago, the health of people who lost their coverage declined dramatically. In 1988, the wealthy, well-insured residents of Beverly Hills had one internist for every 566 people; the poor, ill-insured residents of nearby Compton had one internist for every 19,422 people.

"We've been sucked into believing that if we have a national health program, we're going to have rationing," says Dr. Philip Caper of Dartmouth. "The answer is, we have rationing already. Ask people who lost their health insurance or can't get a bone-marrow transplant because they're on Medicaid. If that isn't rationing, what is?"

Hospitals that serve the poor and uninsured are suffering also. The success of private hospitals in attracting well-insured patients has put an increasing burden on the public and not-for-profit hospitals still willing (or required) to accept all comers. A 1990 survey of 277 public and teaching hospitals found that 38 percent sometimes held patients overnight in the emergency room because no regular beds were available; 40 percent had turned away ambulances because of overcrowding.

Hospitals in California have even shut down their trauma centers as a way of barring the door against uninsured patients. "Hospitals find themselves jockeying for geography," says Bettina Kurowski, a vice-president of St. Joseph Medical Center in Burbank, which closed its trauma center when its annual losses hit $1.5 million and threatened the financial survival of the hospital as a whole. "If you can be promised service areas that include freeways and therefore get trauma cases covered by auto insurance, you can break even. If you can't include freeways, mostly you get penetrating [gunshot and stab-wound] trauma, and those patients by and large don't have insurance."

RED TAPE AND RED INK

Ultimately, our cumbersome, inequitable system of reimbursement raises the costs for all of us—insured and uninsured alike—and causes problems for physicians as well. "In order to preserve the mirage of a private system, we've created the most bureaucratic, regulated system of any in the world," says David Mechanic, director of the Institute on Health Care Policy at Rutgers University.

A key characteristic of the U.S. system is its obsession with making sure that patients get only what their insurance entitles them to, and nothing more. That means, for instance, that hospitals must keep meticulous track of everything used by a particular patient, down to individual gauze sponges or aspirin tablets, thus adding to administrative costs. More important, the burden of dealing with multiple forms from a huge number of insurance companies requires a lot of clerical time and energy.

Increasingly, too, doctors and hospitals have to answer to government and private review panels that evaluate many aspects of the care they offer. Government reviewers work to ensure that Medicare and Medicaid patients are not being undertreated, while private insurers want to make sure that their patients are not overtreated by doctors and hospitals.

On average, U.S. hospitals spend fully 20 percent of their budgets on billing administration, compared to only 9 percent in Canadian hospitals. To run a health plan covering 25 million people, Canada employs fewer administrators than Massachusetts Blue Cross, which covers 2.7 million.

More than 1,200 private health insurance companies add to our national red tape by the necessary maintenance of their underwriting, marketing, and administrative staffs. This overhead consumed an average 14 cents out of every premium dollar in

---

"In order to preserve the mirage of a private system, we've created the most bureaucratic, regulated system of any in the world."

1990, according to the Health Care Financing Administration.

Private physicians, too, have been forced to hire extra office help to cope with the ever-enlarging demands of third-party review, regulations, and paperwork. Drs. David Himmelstein and Steffie Woolhandler, internists at Harvard Medical School who are prominent critics of the U.S. health care system, have calculated that the average office-based U.S. physician employs twice as many clerical and managerial workers as the average Canadian doctor. Bureaucracy has become so intrusive that doctors have developed a name for it: the "hassle factor." Dishonest physicians have also taken advantage of this morass to bilk insurance companies. According to the

47

General Accounting Office report: "This complex system itself becomes an impediment to detecting fraud and abuse. . . . a physician who bills for more office visits than can reasonably be performed in a day, for example, may not be detected if the billing is split among several payers."

Drs. Woolhandler and Himmelstein, who favor a Canadian-style system, have calculated that about 20 percent of U.S. health care spending goes for administrative costs: insurance overhead, hospital and nursing administration, and physicians' overhead and billing expenses. Not surprisingly, the private health insurance industry says this estimate is too high. However, industry representatives decline to offer their own figure.

Universal coverage and uniform fee schedules enable other countries to avoid most of the administrative expense of the U.S. system. The single-payer Canadian system, where all health care costs are ultimately paid by the government, devotes about 10 percent of expenditures to administration. The General Accounting Office calculates that if the United States were to adopt a single-payer Canadian-style system, we would save about $70 billion a year in insurance overhead and the administrative costs to doctors and hospitals.

THE $200-BILLION BOTTOM LINE

To date, no one has come up with a comprehensive price tag for unnecessary medical care, overpriced procedures, and inefficient administration in the U.S. health care system. After extensive review of the literature, however, we believe that *$200 billion* is a conservative estimate of the amount the health care system will waste this year. Of the $817 billion projected to be spent this year, about one-fifth, or $163 billion, will go for administrative costs. Except for a fraction of a percent spent on research, the rest, roughly $650 billion, will go to actual patient care. (Physician and hospital services together make up most of that total, with the rest going to dentists, nursing homes, drugs, and various other expenses.)

Many researchers have now attempted to quantify the rate at which specific procedures are used unnecessarily. Twenty percent represents a rough average of the rates found in major studies and is a figure that several leading researchers in this field told us was a good approximation for the rate of unnecessary care. By our estimates, then, at least 20 percent of that $650 billion, or *$130 billion*, will be spent on procedures and services that are clearly unnecessary.

Twenty percent also seems to be a conservative estimate of the rate of unnecessary hospital days, even though changes in Medicare and private insurance policies make it difficult to estimate that number precisely.

As Dr. John Wennberg of Dartmouth and his colleagues have demonstrated repeatedly, the rate at which physicians use a given procedure can vary four- or fivefold between one location and another. The supply of hospitals and physicians also varies greatly. Except in extreme cases where people lack

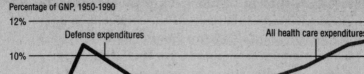

HEALTH VS. EDUCATION VS. DEFENSE

Shifting shares Forty years ago, the U.S. spent about the same on health as on national defense, which was about twice the amount spent on education. Today, education and defense spending are about even, while health outlays take more of the GNP than the other two put together.

Percentage of GNP, 1950-1990

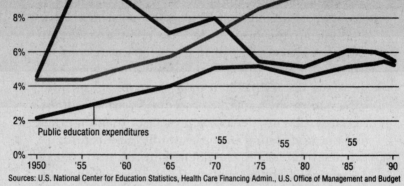

Defense expenditures

All health care expenditures

Public education expenditures

'55   '55   '55

12% 10% 8% 6% 4% 2% 0%

1950 '55 '60 '65 '70 '75 '80 '85 '90

Sources: U.S. National Center for Education Statistics, Health Care Financing Admin., U.S. Office of Management and Budget

access to basic medical care, people living in low-use or low-supply areas seem to be just as healthy as those in high-use or high-supply areas.

Dr. Wennberg and his colleagues argue that areas with abundant doctors and hospitals could provide significantly fewer health care services without harmful consequences. Similarly, the high rates of procedures done in many areas could be cut back without overall harm. This sort of adjustment happens automatically, they note, in industrialized countries that control costs by capping the amount of money available for health care.

If overuse of medical services wastes $130 billion a

year, administrative inefficiency wastes another *$70 billion*. Projecting from 1991 estimates by the General Accounting Office, the nation could save roughly $70 billion this year by switching from our fragmented and inefficient insurance system to a single-payer system, one in which all citizens receive health care from private doctors and hospitals that are paid by a single insurance entity. The savings would come roughly equally from insurance company overhead and hospital and administrative costs.

Adding those two figures together—$130 billion plus $70 billion—gives an estimate of $200 billion for the annual waste in the U.S. health care system. Still, this estimate leaves out several important elements: physicians' fees and the cost of technology, drugs, and procedures. If those costs were brought into line with reimbursement standards in other countries, the savings would be greater.

Moreover, we have not added in the cost of outright fraud, a factor that the General Accounting Office estimates could eat up a full 10 percent of the total health care budget. Some physicians cheat the system by ordering unnecessary tests and procedures, a type of fraud that is included in our estimates of unnecessary care. Other types of fraud, however, would not have been caught in the studies done on unnecessary care. These include billing for services never rendered, falsifying reimbursement codes to collect more than the usual payment for a service, and submitting inflated bills for supplies and devices.

Granted, devising a totally efficient system would be difficult, if not impossible, to accomplish. Howev-

51

er, there is more than enough excess spending in our current system to take care of the roughly 14 percent of the population who are not currently covered by any public or private insurance plan.

ADVICE TO CONSUMERS: MEDICAL RED FLAGS

As long as our medical system remains organized the way it is now, individual consumers will have little direct control over medical costs. Indeed, it's difficult for the average patient even to learn in advance what a doctor or hospital plans to charge for a visit or procedure. In Florida, hospitals have gone to court to resist being forced to reveal their prices. Nor can individuals exercise much control over what is done to them. As we have seen, medicine is a complex field with choices so numerous and unclear that doctors themselves have difficulty with them.

There is, however, one limited area in which consumers can at least raise some questions: the possibility of being offered unnecessary or overpriced treatments. Certain treatments, by virtue of their cost or ubiquity, have attracted special attention from the growing army of consultants, utilization review firms, and researchers looking for unnecessary care. These treatments, listed below, are hardly the only instances of unnecessary care in the system. Neither, of course, does a procedure's presence on the list mean that it is always used unnecessarily, or even that that is usually the case.

Nevertheless, if your physician suggests that you have one of these procedures, you would be well

advised to think twice. You might want to seek a second opinion, if possible, or question your doctor closely on alternatives to the suggested treatment.

Cesarean section. About one in four U.S. births is completed surgically, a rate that may be twice the ideal. In this country, obstetricians routinely perform cesareans when the baby is breech, or for the vaguely defined diagnoses of "prolonged labor" or "fetal distress." Hospitals that have systematically set out to eliminate unnecessary cesareans have cut their rate at least in half without any apparent risk to mothers or babies.

In recent years, the electronic fetal monitor, a device for tracking the fetal heart rate during labor, has come to be used routinely in American hospitals and has contributed to the high cesarean-section rate. Since abnormal fetal heart rates are associated with oxygen deprivation, it was assumed that prompt, automatic detection would enable doctors to intervene early enough to prevent fetal brain damage—for example, by performing a cesarean section on the mother.

But since the fetal monitor's introduction, no fewer than nine comparative studies, involving tens of thousands of women, have failed to demonstrate the hoped-for benefit. Monitored women do have a higher rate of cesarean sections and other costly interventions. But their babies fare no better than those of women monitored by the traditional means, in which a nurse simply checks the fetal heartbeat periodically with a stethoscope.

Hysterectomy. After cesarean section, this is the second most common major surgery in the United States. Value Health Sciences, a firm that applies the Rand Corporation's methodology for insurance industry clients, calls 27 percent of hysterectomies unnecessary, the highest percentage of all procedures it evaluates. Rates of hysterectomy also vary greatly throughout the country, an indication that physician practice and preference play as much of a role as objective need in the decision to perform the operation. Many gynecologists still routinely recommend hysterectomy for fibroids, uterine prolapse, and heavy bleeding; alternative treatments are available for all three conditions.

Back surgery. Value Health Sciences has reported that 14 percent of proposed laminectomies, the most common type of back surgery, are unnecessary. Occasionally, some material from a ruptured disc will press on spinal nerves and cause disabling or painful symptoms that require surgical correction, says Dr. Charles Fager, a neurosurgeon at the Lahey Clinic in Burlington, Mass. But usually, back pain yields to bed rest, the passage of time, physical therapy, or a combination thereof. "I only operate on one out of every 25 or 30 people I see," says Dr. Fager. Some surgeons are not as finicky. Dr. John Wennberg of Dartmouth Medical School has traced sudden "epidemics" of back surgery to the arrival of a new neurosurgeon in a locality.

Magnetic resonance imaging. This powerful new imaging technique, which produces detailed

pictures of internal organs without exposing the patient to radiation, is still so new that doctors are working out its best uses. In the process, they inevitably use it when they have no need to. Some groups of physicians have invested in MRI machines, creating the added temptation to profit by referring their patients for the test. Also, because MRI is virtually risk-free, it's especially likely to be overused as a defensive measure.

Experts stress that MRI procedures, which cost about $1,000 apiece, should be ordered only when a patient's symptoms suggest he or she may have a condition that cannot be diagnosed definitively in any other way.

Prostate surgery. Dr. Wennberg and his colleagues at Dartmouth have shown that surgery for noncancerous enlargement of the prostate is among the most variable of procedures. They have also looked closely at what happens to men who get the surgery and those who do not. For many men, medical therapy can relieve symptoms. For others, putting off surgery is not particularly dangerous, though the urinary obstruction caused by the condition can be uncomfortable. When patients in a health maintenance organization were fully informed in advance of the risks and benefits of surgery, in a study that Dr. Wennberg designed, 80 percent of men with severe urinary symptoms chose to postpone the operation.

Clot-busting drugs. These drugs, when administered within four to six hours of the onset of a heart attack, can break up the blood clot blocking the coro-

nary artery and thus greatly reduce the damage to the heart muscle. The largest comparative study done to date, of 41,000 patients worldwide, has found that all currently available clot-busting drugs are about equally effective in preventing fatal heart attacks. But one, streptokinase, has the lowest incidence of the most dangerous side effect, cerebral hemorrhage.

Of the two drugs used in the United States, streptokinase also happens to be by far the cheaper—about $200 per dose compared to $2,000 per dose for its genetically engineered competitor, tissue plasminogen activator (TPA). Nevertheless, TPA commands a majority of the U.S. market, apparently thanks to aggressive marketing by its manufacturer, Genentech.

For a person having a first heart attack, there is no reason to be treated with the more costly drug. Second treatments with streptokinase, however, are unsafe, since the first treatment can set up the mechanism for an allergic response to any future injection.

That worked well for a while. More workers had health insurance, and their coverage broadened to include doctors' visits, prescription drugs, and even treatment for mental illness. But now the system stitched together over the last 45 years is unraveling, and people are being deprived of needed health care.

THE PLIGHT OF THE UNINSURED

People without health insurance include men and women who work for small businesses, the self-employed, part-time workers, young people just starting their careers, the disabled, and those taking early retirement who are still too young for Medicare. Many of the uninsured are also poor. Medicaid, the federal and state program that covers the medical expenses for the indigent, currently pays the bills for only 40 percent of the nation's poor.

People without health insurance may not get medical care. Currently, 1 million families each year try to obtain care when they are sick, but find they cannot afford it.

Unfortunately, too, others without insurance postpone treatment when they are sick. If they are not ill, people without insurance postpone preventive care until more costly treatment is necessary—or until it's too late.

Two-thirds of all people with hypertension, or high blood pressure, fail to have their disease treated, largely because they cannot afford the medications. Half of those with hypertension have not seen a doctor within the past year. A 1990 poll found that the proportion of Americans going to doctors in any one month for any reason had fallen to a 15-year low.

Women are particularly at risk. Uninsured women are much less likely than insured women to have screening tests for breast and cervical cancer or for glaucoma. If they are pregnant, they often do without prenatal care. Some 5 million women between the ages of 15 and 44 are covered by private health insurance policies that do not include coverage for maternity care.

"The proportion of Americans going to doctors in any one month for any reason has fallen to a 15-year low."

Lack of prenatal care translates into babies who are too small when they are born and babies who die soon after birth. The United States trails 23 other nations in the percentage of babies born with an adequate birth weight and ranks 22nd in the rate of infant mortality, behind such countries as Spain and Singapore.

SHIFTING THE COST

Each year thousands of people are dumped into emergency rooms of public hospitals because private hospitals do not want patients who cannot pay. In 1989, unpaid hospital bills totaled $10 billion, up 7 percent from the previous year. To recoup the costs of unpaid care, hospitals and doctors simply raise their fees to those who do pay: primarily, the private insurance carriers and patients who foot almost 60 percent of the nation's medical bill.

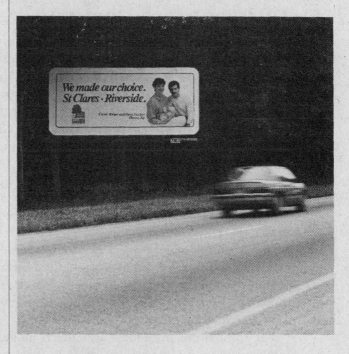

Hospitals in some parts of the country advertise to fill their beds, partly because of insurance company rules requiring that more procedures be done on an outpatient basis.

Such cost shifting drives up the price of insurance, resulting in even more people who cannot afford coverage. In New Jersey, for example, every hospital bill now carries a 19-percent surcharge, reflecting the hospital revenue lost to unpaid bills. That feeds into higher insurance premiums.

Cost shifting accounts for about one-third of the increase in insurance premiums, which are rising at a rate of about 20 percent a year. The cost of medical care, which is increasing two to three times faster than the rate of inflation, is responsible for the rest.

UNAFFORDABLE PREMIUMS

The higher the price tag for insurance, the greater the number of people who go without it. Firms with fewer than 100 workers employ about one-third of the U.S. work force, but only about half of those small businesses offer health insurance to their employees. Small-business owners say they have enough trouble staying afloat without assuming the heavy burden of health insurance premiums.

Even when employers do offer coverage, not all their employees take it. In 1987, 25 percent of the uninsured worked for very large employers, most of whom offered insurance.

People who want coverage and must buy it on their own have little choice but to pay what the insurance company demands. In many instances, that can mean thousands of dollars each year. And premiums continue to rise dramatically.

The spiraling of premiums also affects millions of the insured whose employers provide their health insurance. One major employee benefits survey found that employers now spend about $3,600 annually to cover each employee. In many cases the employers are shifting some of those ever-increasing costs to their workers by requiring them to pay a greater share of the premium and a larger portion of their medical expenses through higher deductibles and copayments.

In 1986, Foster and Higgins, a benefits consulting firm, found that 59 percent of employers paid the full premium for their individual workers. By 1991, that figure was down to 45 percent. In 1986, 30 percent of employers paid the full premium for family coverage; in 1991 the figure was 24 percent.

More than half of employers try to trim their insurance outlays by self-insuring. They invest the premiums they would otherwise spend on insurance and pay employees' claims directly when they arise.

The Employee Retirement Income Security Act (ERISA) exempts these self-insured plans from state-insurance regulations meant to protect consumers. For example, employers may not have to offer certain coverages, such as care for newborn children, or to provide for continuation of coverage when employees leave.

Employers hire a third-party administrator, or TPA, to handle the claims. Because the TPA may be the local Blue Cross and Blue Shield plan, employees may think that Blue Cross (or some other insurance company) is actually underwriting their coverage. Little do they know that the loopholes created by ERISA can leave them without any health insurance coverage if things go wrong. If the employer goes out of business or stops providing coverage, employees may be out of luck.

CLINGING TO COVERAGE

Millions of Americans have yet to lose their insurance, but could at any time be the victims of an insurance company's business practices. As health care providers continually raise their fees and pass on the higher cost of medical care to insurance companies, the companies respond by insuring fewer people. People who must buy coverage on their own and workers in small firms feel this pinch the hardest.

Insurance companies are not charities. Their goal is to make a profit, and they can increase their odds of success by insuring people who are unlikely to have health problems. Competition among carriers for the healthiest risks has become cutthroat.

In large businesses with many employees, it scarcely matters if some employees have serious medical conditions. The risk they pose can easily be spread among the healthy workers. But in a small group with few employees, insurance companies cannot always collect enough in premiums to pay for the claims of those who are sick. So the rules for insuring workers in small businesses are more rigorous.

Insurers use a controversial scheme to insulate themselves from risk. They offer to insure employees in a small firm (usually those with fewer than 25 workers) at a "low-ball" premium for at least the first year. If members of the group experience costly health problems in the second and third years, the carrier tosses the firm into a pool with other groups whose health care costs are high and jacks up its premiums as much as 200 percent.

By placing firms into several "rate tiers," insurance companies can bid for the healthiest groups with rock-bottom premiums. But employers and their employees who have had serious health problems are stuck with their present insurance carrier; they cannot move to another, because no other company is likely to take them at any premium. Worse, the present carrier may decide not to renew the group's coverage, forcing employers and employees to find other insurance. And that may be impossible.

NO COVERAGE FOR THE SICK

Companies insuring small groups require employees and their dependents to meet tough health requirements, just as they do for individuals buying policies on their own. No carrier wants to insure employees and dependents who have had heart attacks or cancer. They will either exclude them from the policy or decline to insure the group altogether. Sometimes a single employee with a serious disease is enough to earn a rejection slip for the whole group.

Increasingly, insurance companies are turning down people with far less serious health conditions than cancer or heart disease, excluding everyone except those in perfect or near-perfect health. "We don't want to buy a claim," is how one company official puts it.

A CASE OF THE BLUES

Sick people cannot buy a policy from Blue Cross and Blue Shield of Kentucky, whose plan evaluates an applicant's health and rejects those with such afflictions as cancer, heart disease, emphysema, and AIDS.

Competition from commercial carriers has forced the plan to turn sick people away in order to keep its premiums affordable and attract new customers. At one time, Kentucky's Blue Cross and Blue Shield sold as much as 90 percent of all health insurance in the state. Today it sells just 34 percent.

"Increasingly, insurance companies are turning down people with far less serious health conditions than cancer or heart disease, excluding everyone except those in perfect or near-perfect health."

The Kentucky plan, typical of many Blue Cross and Blue Shield organizations today, is a far cry from what such plans used to be. Founded by organized medicine in the 1930s, Blue Cross (and later Blue Shield) had two missions. The first was to make sure hospitals and doctors got paid. The second was to provide health insurance for the greatest number of people.

For years, the "Blues" had a virtual insurance monopoly. In some places, they were so powerful that they were able to negotiate large discounts from hospitals and use the savings to carry out their mission of community service. For example, Blue Cross subsidized such money losers as individual health policies for the sick and Medicare-supplement coverage for the elderly.

As nonprofit organizations, the Blues had certain privileges. They paid no federal income taxes and, in many states, no taxes on the premiums they collected.

"Community rating" was once the Blues' trademark. All members of the community—large employer groups, small employer groups, and individuals buying policies on their own—were in the same risk pool. They paid the same rates regardless of their age and sex, where they lived, or how sick they were.

That all began to change in the 1960s. Commercial insurers started skimming the best risks from the Blue Cross pool by offering lower premiums than the Blues charged. As large groups and then small ones took out cheaper policies with commercial carriers, the Blues increasingly found themselves covering people with health problems the commercial carriers did not want. As healthy people deserted the pool, the Blues had little choice but to raise premiums higher and higher to cover the claims made by the sick people who remained.

In many areas, the plans also saw their hospital discounts whittled away. Some states now mandate smaller discounts and allow all insurers to receive them.

Blue Cross and Blue Shield of Kentucky, for example, is not entitled to a hospital discount any larger than that of its commercial competitors. And it does not subsidize individual health coverage (other than conversion policies) out of the profits from other lines of business. At the suggestion of insurance regulators, it abandoned community rating a few years ago in favor of the kind of pricing used by commercial insurers.

Most Blue Cross and Blue Shield plans now resemble Kentucky's. Many have become mutual insurance companies. They have lost their tax exemption from the federal government, and they no longer try to provide coverage for everyone. Less than one-third still take all comers for health insurance. Of the 37 state regulators responding to a 1989 Consumers Union survey, only nine considered their local Blue Cross and Blue Shield plan an insurer of last resort.

Some Blue Cross and Blue Shield plans, mostly in the Northeast, still cling to the old mission. But even for them, holding on is increasingly difficult. In New York, a person can always get health insurance from Empire Blue Cross / Blue Shield, no matter how sick. It won't be the top-of-the-line policy, but it will provide some coverage. Empire, which still uses community rates, can sell insurance even to people with terminal illnesses because their policies are heavily subsidized from premiums paid by large employer groups and from the savings obtained by discounts from New York hospitals.

Even so, Empire officials say that over the last four years some 400,000 people have left the pool, either going with commercial carriers or doing without coverage altogether. The plan lost $150 million in 1991 covering the claims of the sick people who remain. In 1992, the New York legislature passed a law requiring *all* insurers—including commercial carriers—to sell policies to all applicants at community rates. Even so, Empire says it will need rate increases of 20 percent or more over the next three years to restore its financial health.

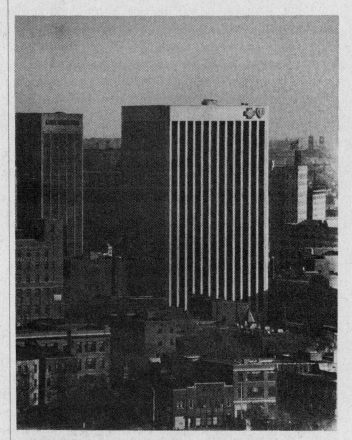

Empire Blue Cross/ Blue Shield in New York City towers over its East Side neighborhood, but its stature as an insurer has weakened.

ADVICE TO CONSUMERS: SHOPPING FOR A PLAN

If you lose your health insurance coverage for any reason, you can remain uninsured and take your chances, or you can venture into the marketplace for an individual policy. Be forewarned: You will not find a buyer's market. And even if your health is good, you may have few options. And before plunking down $2,000 or $3,000 for coverage, you will need to know a little about how these policies work.

There are three basic kinds of health coverage:

- Major-medical policies. These are the most comprehensive, covering both hospital stays and physicians' services in and out of the hospital.
- Hospital-surgical policies. These cover hospital services and surgical procedures only.
- Hospital-indemnity and dread-disease policies. These policies are vastly inferior to the other two types and offer very limited benefits.

WHAT'S COVERED

Major-medical policies typically pay for most hospital services, including room and board; operating and recovery rooms; nursing care; and treatment in intensive-care units, emergency rooms, and outpatient facilities. They also pick up the tab for lab tests, X-rays, anesthesia, medical supplies, ambulance services, and physicians' office visits. Most pay for prescription drugs and cover confinements in skilled-nursing facilities, if necessary, following a hospital stay.

Some policies, however, do not pay for assistant surgeons or for stand-by surgeons. Others will not cover emergency treatment, unless the policyholder is admitted directly to the hospital; this practice discourages the use of emergency rooms for routine treatment. Still others limit the number of times they will pay for doctors' visits in the hospital. Even a comprehensive policy may pay for only one visit each day.

Hospital-surgical policies cover hospital room and board, often for a specified number of days; treatment in intensive-care and outpatient facilities; medical supplies; surgeon's fees; diagnostic tests relating to an operation; some radiation and chemotherapy; and sometimes second opinions. But they cover almost no expenses incurred outside a hospital. They will not pay for a doctor's office visit to check on a persistent cough, to have your child's cast removed, or for any medical condition that does not require hospitalization. Most do not cover prescription drugs that you may need outside a hospital.

Generally, both major-medical and hospital-surgical policies pay for 30 days of inpatient treatment for mental illness and substance abuse. Some major-medical policies cover outpatient treatment as well. If they do, insurers limit the number of visits per year or even the dollar amount of their payments.

Maternity benefits. Most major-medical and hospital-surgical policies pay for expenses arising from pregnancy complications. But with the exception of some Blue Cross and Blue Shield plans, they usually do not cover routine prenatal care or routine deliveries.

If you want coverage for that, you have to buy a

separate rider, and at some companies, you need to decide on the rider the day you take out the policy. Some carriers will not let you buy the rider later (on the grounds that you will probably use the coverage, sticking them with a claim). Many major-medical and hospital-surgical policies offer no riders for routine maternity care, period.

Riders will pay up to a maximum benefit that policyholders select, usually $500, $1,000, $2,000, or $2,500. Rarely do they cover the full cost of a normal delivery.

Another drawback is that companies do not pay the full benefit during the first two years the policy is in force. A policyholder who becomes pregnant may receive only 50 or 60 percent of the benefit in the first year and 75 percent in the second year. Not until the third year are full benefits paid.

WHAT'S NOT COVERED

Both major-medical and hospital-surgical policies cover only medically necessary care. Do not count on them to pay for routine physicals or other preventive services. (Some of them, however, cover Pap smears, mammography, and well-child care.) Neither do they pay for cosmetic surgery, fertility treatment, dental care, hearing aids, surgical treatment of obesity, treatment for self-inflicted injuries, or procedures that are considered experimental.

Insurance companies compute the amount of your reimbursement check according to their own complex formulas. The amount may be higher or lower depending on the following.

Eligible expenses. When you submit a bill for a service covered by a major-medical policy, the insurer compares it with the amount it normally pays for that service. If the charge is lower than what the company determines is "usual," "customary," "reasonable," or "common," then the entire bill is eligible for reimbursement. If it is greater, the carrier will consider only a portion of it.

What portion the company considers differs among insurers. Each company sets its reimbursement level based on physicians' charges for services and procedures in your area. One company might choose to reimburse policyholders based on the charge that represents the 90th percentile for a given procedure or service. Another might choose the 75th percentile. (For hospital services, companies pay either the hospital's posted charge, the hospital's cost, or a negotiated fee.)

Obviously, the higher the reimbursement standard, the more you will receive. Unfortunately, policies rarely spell that out.

Some hospital-surgical policies work differently, paying up to a maximum amount for each covered procedure or service listed in the policy. There is usually one fee schedule for hospital room and board, one for surgeon's fees, another for outpatient services, and a maximum amount the policy will pay for all other hospital services. This is the equivalent of a hospital-surgical policy's eligible charge. Amounts paid by hospital-surgical policies usually fall far short of the actual charges.

Coinsurance. Once the insurer determines how much of your bill it will consider, it still pays only a portion. You pay the rest. That is called "coinsurance."

Most major-medical policies pay 80 percent of eligible expenses, leaving policyholders to pay the remaining 20 percent, plus that part of the cost not covered at all. (A few major-medical policies require a smaller coinsurance payment, or none at all, while others may have copayments of as much as 50 percent.)

Suppose a physician charges $3,000 for an angioplasty (a cardiac procedure), but the carrier considers only $2,610 as an eligible expense. If the insurer pays 80 percent, the policyholder will receive $2,088 (80 percent of $2,610). He or she will then have to pay the remaining 20 percent, or $522, plus the $390 that's not eligible for reimbursement.

With some policies from Blue Cross and Blue Shield, a policyholder who used a "participating physician" would pay less. Participating physicians agree not to bill patients in excess of what Blue Cross and Blue Shield pays. This can be a significant advantage.

Coinsurance maximums. Most policies specify a maximum dollar amount of coinsurance, typically $1,000 (but it can be as much as $2,500 or $5,000), that policyholders must pay annually. After they have reached that amount, the carrier pays 100 percent of all additional, eligible medical expenses.

A few policies tie coinsurance maximums to the size

of the deductible you select. The higher the deductible, the lower the maximum.

Several policies give a break to families. Usually two members must each pay the maximum coinsurance amount. The company will then pay 100 percent of all eligible expenses for other members who have not reached their maximums.

Lifetime maximums. Most major-medical and hospital-surgical policies cap the benefits they will pay over a lifetime at $1 million or sometimes $2 million. A few have no cap, and others have a separate lifetime maximum for each illness or injury.

A company will sometimes give new lifetime benefits to policyholders who have generated enough claims to reach their lifetime cap. This is an important feature if the cap is low.

Deductibles. Most companies require policyholders to satisfy deductibles each year before benefits are paid. (Some hospital-surgical policies have no deductibles.) Deductibles can be as low as $100 or as high as $20,000. That means a policyholder must pay the first $100 (or $20,000) of expenses before the company pays any benefits. Obviously, a $20,000 deductible buys only catastrophic protection.

Sometimes a policy links the deductible to an illness or health condition; you would have to satisfy the deductible with each new illness. If the deductible is large and you have several different illnesses, you may never collect any benefits.

Some companies no longer offer low deductibles.

"If somebody can afford to buy our product, he can afford a $1,000 deductible," said John Hartnedy, the chief actuary at Golden Rule. "You don't want first-dollar coverage. It may cost $80 to take care of a $50 bill."

As with most insurance, the higher the deductible, the lower the premium. Sometimes, for a small extra premium, companies will waive the deductible or a portion of it if you are injured in an accident.

ARE YOU INSURABLE?

People who have medical problems, however minor, are second-class citizens in the world of health insurance. Virtually no commercial carriers and only a handful of Blue Cross and Blue Shield plans will sell policies to anyone who has had heart disease, internal cancer, diabetes, strokes, adrenal disorders, epilepsy, or ulcerative colitis. Treatment for alcohol and substance abuse, depression, or even visits to a marriage counselor can also mean a rejection.

If you have less serious conditions, you may get coverage, but on unfavorable terms. Conditions that usually affect one part of the body are candidates for "exclusion riders"—that is, companies will offer a policy, but exclude coverage for those conditions or that body part, either for a short period or for as long as the policy is in force. If you have had a recent knee operation, glaucoma, migraine headaches, varicose veins, arthritis, a cesarean delivery, or if your child suffers from chronic ear infections, your policy will probably carry an exclusion rider. "Any condition that would produce an immediate claim would be

Can You Renew?

Few companies will guarantee to renew your coverage. Most policies are "conditionally renewable": The company can refuse to renew your policy only if it also refuses to renew all other similar policies in your state. You have some protection because the company cannot single you out for cancellation. Still, you can lose your coverage. Some insurance companies use conditionally renewable policies as a lever to force insurance regulators to grant the rate increases those companies want.

A few policies are "optionally renewable." A company can opt not to renew your insurance whether or not it renews coverage for others who have the same policy. Many companies also give themselves the option of not renewing if they find you have another policy that is similar.

ridered out," said Frank Fugiel, a vice president at Washington National.

If you have a medical condition that affects your general health—for example, you are significantly overweight or have high blood pressure—you may get coverage, but at a price 15 to 100 percent higher than the standard premium.

Insurers, however, are not restrictive in identical ways. One may exclude coverage for your eyes if you had a cataract operation a year ago, while another may permit it. If you suffered from migraine headaches in the past but have had no treatment for the last two years, some companies will cover future migraine treatment, while some will issue a policy that excludes migraine treatment.

Even if your health is perfect, you still may be a less-than-perfect risk. In avoiding applicants who are likely to file claims, insurance companies blackball people in certain occupations. Some companies have long lists of jobs that are unacceptable, either for an individual policy or for a policy sold to employees in small firms. Chances are, the insurance company will not cover you if it considers your work hazardous or if people in your profession are more likely to file claims or switch jobs frequently.

BETTER OFF AT THE BLUES?

Historically, most Blue Cross and Blue Shield plans took all comers for individual health insurance, offering "open-enrollment" policies that anyone could buy. Even if your health was bad, you could count on getting a policy from the Blues.

Today, only a minority of Blue Cross and Blue Shield plans still make policies available to everyone, and their "open-enrollment" policies may require policyholders to pay a larger portion of their expenses than policies offered to those in good health. Most Blue Cross and Blue Shield organizations now "underwrite," evaluating an applicant's health much the same way their commercial competitors do. They reject people with cancer and heart disease and sometimes issue policies with exclusion riders and higher premiums.

It's hard to say whether you will have an easier time buying coverage from the Blues than from commercial insurers. Blue Cross plans that do not exclude health conditions or charge higher premiums for them may simply refuse to sell you a policy. On the other hand, a Blue Cross plan might be more lenient than a commercial insurer.

If you get a policy from Blue Cross and Blue Shield or a commercial insurer, you still may have to wait a year or two to be covered for medical conditions you already have. Most policies say that a pre-existing condition is one for which a policyholder has received treatment or for which a reasonably prudent person should have sought treatment during the previous two years. Some policies have shorter or longer "look-back" periods.

To encourage applicants to reveal all their medical conditions, some companies waive their usual waiting periods if you have disclosed all your health problems, provided that the company is willing to accept you and not exclude coverage for those conditions.

WHAT POLICIES COST

The premiums you pay are based on your age, your sex, and where you live. Older people pay higher premiums than younger, and women higher than men. A few Blue Cross plans still use community rates, charging everyone the same premium regardless of their age or where they live. Other things being equal, older people are usually better off at a company using community rates.

With most policies, premiums increase as you get older. If you buy a policy at age 40, expect the premium to increase when you turn 45.

In addition to age-related increases, the rising cost of medical care also pushes up premiums every year or two. In recent years, premiums for some policies have risen as much as 40 or 50 percent in a single year.

As a sales gimmick, some companies use a pricing scheme that gives policyholders a deceptively low premium the first year and very high premiums in later years. When a company that uses so-called select and ultimate rates accepts you for coverage, it knows you are in good health and charges a low (select) premium to reflect the fact that you are not likely to file claims in the immediate future. But as the years go on, and as you make claims, the company will jack up the premium to the highest (ultimate) level.

Companies that do not use select and ultimate rates spread the anticipated costs of your claims over all the years you own the policy, so your premiums will be more stable. If you buy from a company using select and ultimate rates, you may face premium increases that you cannot afford.

State insurance regulators do not require insurers to disclose whether they use select and ultimate rates, so it's a good idea to ask whether a company you are considering uses such rates and to avoid such policies, especially if you plan to keep the coverage for several years.

INSURANCE POLICIES TO AVOID

The worst buys in health insurance are hospital-indemnity policies and dread-disease policies. Hospital-indemnity policies pay a fixed amount each day you are in the hospital. Dread-disease policies pay benefits only if you contract cancer or some other specified illness.

"The worst buys in health insurance are hospital-indemnity policies and dread-disease policies."

The hospital-indemnity deal is simple and understandable. You get a fixed dollar amount for each day you spend in the hospital. No complicated deductibles or coinsurance. The trouble is, the fixed benefit is skimpy to start with and grows less valuable with each passing year. Even the most generous hospital-indemnity plans will barely dent the average hospital bill. Furthermore, to collect the high benefits touted by some of the ads, you need to be hospitalized as long as a month—an unlikely prospect, since the average stay is only about seven days. Finally, the benefit does not change. In time, inflation in hospital and medical costs inevitably shrinks its value. Dread-disease policies offer similarly inadequate benefits.

Companies also sell riders to cover such dread diseases as smallpox, polio, rabies, diphtheria, and typhoid fever. It's hard to understand why anyone would buy them, since these diseases are now extremely rare.

Compared to other health coverages, these types of insurance are cheap. Insurers usually issue hospital-indemnity policies to all applicants, whether or not they are in good health. But the policies often require a waiting period before covering policyholders for preexisting health conditions.

Most companies selling cancer insurance will not issue policies to people who already have cancer. Nor do they usually pay benefits to anyone who is diagnosed as having the disease before the policy has been in force for 30 days.

These policies are no substitute for comprehensive health coverage. The price is low, but so are the benefits. With a dread-disease policy, you are gambling that you will contract one of the covered diseases. If you never do, the policy will be useless. Companies often market these policies as a supplement to other insurance. But we do not recommend them even for that. The $300, $400, or $500 you would spend for inferior coverage may equal the difference in premium between a skimpy hospital-surgical policy and a more comprehensive major-medical policy. Or it may cover the cost of taking a lower deductible on a good major-medical policy.

THE LAST RESORT: HIGH-RISK POOLS

If you cannot buy health insurance, you have an insurer of last resort if you live in one of the 26 states with a high-risk pool created for the people insurance carriers want to avoid. Similar to the high-risk plans for drivers who have been in automobile accidents, health insurance pools originated in the 1970s as the industry's alternative to national health insurance. But only in the last few years have states begun to get serious about them.

To obtain coverage, you usually must have been a state resident for at least six months (a year in some states) and have received a rejection notice from at least one carrier. If a carrier will insure you only at a premium exceeding the price of coverage from the pool, or if the insurance offered you carries exclusion riders, you will also be eligible for a pool policy in most states.

The rules differ from state to state. Some state pools exclude people infected with the HIV virus; some let them in. In some states you cannot get pool coverage if you are eligible for a conversion policy when you leave an employer group, even though the pool policy may be better than the conversion option.

Some states make Medicare-supplement policies available through their pools. That is a boon to the disabled under age 65 who rely on Medicare but who can find no insurance to fill Medicare's gaps.

Pool coverage is similar to that offered by a major-medical policy, although benefits for mental and nervous disorders, organ transplants, and pregnancy may be less comprehensive. You may, however, pay more out-of-pocket than you would with a major-medical policy. Some plans require a high deductible, greater coinsurance, and relatively low lifetime-benefit maximums—$500,000 or even $250,000. Premiums are no bargain, which is not surprising, since policyholders in the pool will almost certainly file claims.

Pool policies provide decent coverage, but they are available only to a fraction of those who need them. It's hard to see how the pools can meet even the existing need. They operate at a loss, despite the high premiums. In most states, losses are covered by assessments against all health insurance carriers doing business in the state. In return, some states relieve insurers from part of their obligation to pay taxes on the premiums they collect.

The 26 states with high-risk pools are California, Colorado, Connecticut, Florida, Georgia, Illinois, Indiana, Iowa, Louisiana, Maine, Minnesota, Mississippi, Missouri, Montana, Nebraska, New Mexico, North Dakota, Oregon, Rhode Island, South Carolina, Tennessee, Texas, Utah, Washington, Wisconsin, and Wyoming. Your state insurance department can tell you how to contact your state's pool.

BEYOND THE GROUP PLAN

If you leave a job, you may have two options for continuing your health insurance, short of shopping for an individual policy on your own. Depending on both the size of the firm you worked for and your state's insurance regulations, you may be able to continue your group coverage for a short time, as provided under the Consolidated Omnibus Budget Reconciliation Act of 1985 (COBRA). Or you may be able to obtain an individual policy through a process known as conversion. Both options, though, will usually cost a lot more than you would spend for group coverage.

Because it is less expensive and generally offers better coverage than a conversion policy, your first line of defense should be COBRA. If you worked for a business with 20 or more employees, COBRA entitles you and your dependents to continued coverage for at least 18 months under your former employer's plan. If you are disabled and eligible for Social Security disability benefits when your employment ends, you can obtain an additional 11 months of coverage, for a total of 29 months.

If you are insured through your spouse's plan at work and your spouse dies, you become divorced or separated, or your spouse becomes eligible for Medicare, COBRA provides for coverage of up to 36 months. COBRA requires that you pay 102 percent of your group insurance premium. If your employer has been paying a portion, you will have to assume that cost in addition to what you were already paying, plus an extra 2 percent for administrative costs. Disabled people who take COBRA coverage must pay as much as 150 percent of the premium for the extra 11 months.

You can lose coverage if you do not pay the premiums, if you become eligible for Medicare, if your employer discontinues health insurance for employees still working there, or if you join another plan. However, if you join another plan and have an existing medical condition for which that plan imposes a waiting period, you can still keep your COBRA benefits until they would normally run out. By that time, your preexisting condition may be covered under the new plan. But you could be without coverage for that condition if your COBRA benefits stop before the waiting period on the new policy is over.

If you work for a company that has self-insured its workers' health coverage, you are entitled to COBRA benefits, even though such plans are normally exempt from other insurance regulations.

If you are not eligible for COBRA because your former firm employs fewer than 20 workers (or is a church organization), you may still have some protection under state laws. If your state provides for "continuation" of benefits, you may be able to stay on your employer's group policy for as little as three months in some states or as long as 18 months in others. (Those benefits are usually not available to workers in self-insured plans.)

Some employers consider COBRA an administrative headache and may offer employees who leave a simpler alternative, such as insurance that covers them only for injuries caused in an accident. Accident-only policies may be tempting because they are cheap—a few hundred dollars a year, compared to a few thousand for COBRA coverage—but unless you are very young, you are much more likely to need coverage for illnesses than for accidents.

After COBRA coverage runs out, or if you are ineligible for it, your next option is to take a conversion
policy or shop for individual coverage (unless, of
course, you are covered under a new employer's
health plan or become eligible for Medicare).

The law states that every employer who normally
offers conversion policies to workers who leave must
also offer them to former employees once their
COBRA benefits run out.

If an insurance company terminates a group plan,
employees may be out of luck. But two-thirds of the
states require insurers that cancel group policies to
offer conversion options to people losing their coverage.

Even when it is offered, conversion coverage is
almost always inferior to what you had under your
group plan. (About half the states require companies
to offer conversion policies with major-medical or
comprehensive benefits.) If you currently have
major-medical coverage, a conversion policy may
provide only hospital-surgical benefits and only pay
up to a fixed amount each day for hospital room and
board and surgical procedures.

While benefits are low, the prices of conversion
policies are high, reflecting the fact that it is mostly
people in poor health who buy this coverage. Despite
those drawbacks, a conversion policy may be your
only option if you have health problems. Insurers
must make these policies available to all applicants
regardless of their health.

If only one member of your family suffers from
some medical condition, you may want to take the

conversion policy for him or her and try to find cheaper, individual coverage for the rest of the family. In some states, a person with health problems may be eligible for coverage from the high-risk pool, although in certain states, if you're eligible for a conversion policy, you cannot have pool coverage.

If you are considering buying an individual policy instead of taking your conversion option when COBRA coverage ends, do your shopping well in advance. The slightest health problem can disqualify you, and it may take time for an insurer to collect your medical records and decide if it's willing to issue coverage. Once your COBRA benefits run out, you have only 31 days in most states to sign up for a conversion policy.

3
IS MANAGED CARE
THE ANSWER?

"HMO members usually receive more benefits for their premiums than patients with traditional insurance do."

More and more workers, urged or even pushed by employers no longer able to pay the enormous increases in health insurance premiums, are trading in their traditional insurance coverage for membership in a health maintenance organization or other so-called managed-care plan.

Enrollment in HMOs, the earliest form of managed care, has doubled since 1985. The first such organizations, Kaiser Permanente in California and the Health Insurance Plan of Greater New York (HIP), sprang up more than 40 years ago as alternatives to traditional, fragmented, fee-for-service medicine. In the early prepaid group-practice plans, as they were known, salaried physicians delivered medical services under one roof for a fixed monthly fee paid by members or their employers. Since the plan received the same amount of money whether members were sick or well, one of its goals was to keep people well by providing preventive services that traditional insurance did not cover. Prepaid group practices also tried to deliver care less expensively by coordinating all treatment, controlling use of hospital services, and limiting referrals to specialists.

The idea of prepaid group practice got a boost in the early 1970s, when the Nixon administration latched onto it as a way to thwart proposals for national health insurance. Coining the term "health maintenance organization," the administration promoted legislation that would give the federal government's seal of approval to groups that met certain standards.

But by then, many HMOs had begun to move away from the ideals of the prepaid group-practice plans. The federal law passed in 1973 allowed organizations that were very different from the older plans to call themselves HMOs.

Today some 550 organizations have adopted the HMO label. Some have been formed by hospitals, some by physician groups, some by entrepreneurs. They still provide health care for their members for a fixed monthly premium. But they range from the restrictive arrangements found in traditional prepaid group plans to loose confederations of doctors whose practices look, feel, and smell like old-fashioned fee-for-service medicine.

Besides the myriad HMOs, a number of look-alikes have appeared that seem like HMOs but often lack the health care management features of the real thing.

THE HMO NETWORK

The foundation of an HMO is the network of doctors and hospitals it has built to provide health care for its members. How carefully they have been chosen can determine the kind of care you will receive.

In constructing a network, an HMO tries to find doctors who will play by the HMO's rules. It may recruit physicians who have admitting privileges at a particular hospital, or it may simply invite all doctors in an area to join. Some networks have only a few doctors. That means either that the HMO was very selective or that many doctors refused to join. Other networks have many doctors, giving members more choice, but making it harder for the HMO to monitor the use of medical services and quality of care.

Choice, however, is a key to member happiness. "One of our strong points is a large panel of doctors—6,000," says Allan Greenberg, chief executive officer of Pilgrim Health Care, one of the top-rated HMOs in the *Consumer Reports* Ratings. Of the *Consumer Reports* readers in Pilgrim's plan who responded to the magazine's annual survey (which included a section on HMOs) about three-quarters were highly satisfied with their doctors.

The process by which HMOs choose doctors, called "credentialing," varies considerably among HMOs. "At some HMOs, all a doctor needs is a license and admitting privileges at a hospital," says Peggy O'Kane, president of the National Committee for Quality Assurance, an HMO accreditation group. Other HMOs look somewhat more deeply into doctors' qualifications. They will check such obvious indicators as license status, malpractice suits, board certification, and whether the doctors keep regular office hours. Sometimes plan officials will visit physicians' offices to look for any obvious deficiencies. Even then, however, the HMO may know little about the quality of a doctor's work.

Once the doctors are chosen, most HMOs then pick hospitals and negotiate a discount with them. In general, the more patients the HMO can send, the greater the discount.

GETTING INTO THE NETWORK

If you join a plan that provides care in health centers, you will have to pick a center, probably one near your home or workplace. If your HMO provides care in doctors' offices, you will have to pick a primary-care doctor from the HMO's directory. (Members who go to health centers may also choose a primary-care doctor.) The primary-care physician is, in effect, the quarterback of the system. He or she decides what health care you will receive and what specialists you will go to. If you need a specialist, he or she will refer you to one in the HMO's network.

The HMO's strategy is to use a primary-care doctor, rather than costlier specialists, to treat common problems. It will be this general practitioner, not an orthopedist, who will treat sprained ankles; the GP, not an otolaryngologist, will treat an earache; and the GP, not a urologist, will take care of urinary tract infections. (In some HMOs, gynecologists, pediatricians, and internists can act as primary-care doctors.)

If you need hospital care, you will have to use one of the hospitals in the HMO's network. In the case of a true emergency, you can go to any hospital but will have to notify the HMO. For emergencies that occur outside the HMO's service area, the HMO will pay for treatment at the nearest hospital if you notify the plan.

What you think of as an emergency may not fit with your HMO's definition of an emergency. One-fifth of the *Consumers Reports* survey respondents who had emergencies and were seen by non-HMO doctors said the plan covered only part of the bill. About 10 percent received no payment at all.

Since an HMO is paid to provide all your medical care, it expects you to stay within the network. If you go outside for treatment, you yourself will usually have to pay the bills.

HOW DOCTORS ARE PAID

In most HMOs, the kind and amount of medical care you receive is directly linked to the way your primary-care doctor is paid. Some HMOs pay doctors salaries and reward them with bonuses at the end of

RATINGS OF HMOs

Listed in order of overall satisfaction index, based on responses to CU's 1991 Annual Questionnaire. Results reflect our respondents' experiences in HMOs from spring 1990 through spring 1991, and may not be representative of the entire HMO population.

Service area. Where our survey respondents for each HMO lived.

Satisfaction index. More than 20,000 respondents rated their HMOs, on a six-point scale ranging from completely satisfied to completely dissatisfied. The index is a summary of those ratings. We had at least 150 responses for each HMO. Had all members been completely satisfied with a plan, its index would have been 100; had all been completely dissatisfied, the index would have been 0. Differences of less than 5 points are not meaningful.

Satisfaction with HMO personnel. Satisfaction with various aspects of HMO's service. These judgments are relative; even the lowest-rated HMOs were judged satisfactory by most of their members. **HMO physician:** Satisfaction with primary-care doctor. Overall, 91 percent were satisfied. **Medical specialists:** Satisfaction with choice of, and access to, specialists. Overall, 86 percent were satisfied. **HMO administration:** Satisfaction with HMO's responsiveness to questions and complaints. Overall, 79 percent were satisfied.

HMO	Service area	Satisfaction index
Heritage National Health Plan	IA, IL, WI, TN	83
Pilgrim Health Care	MA, RI	83
Independent Health	Upstate NY	81
Blue Choice	Upstate NY	80
Preferred Care	Upstate NY	79
Bay State Health Care (now part of Blue Cross Blue Shield of Massachusetts) [1]	MA, RI, NH	79
Physicians Health Plan of Minn. (now Medica Choice)	MN	79
Comprecare	CO	78
Health Alliance Plan	MI	78
Group Health, Inc.	MN, WI	78
Group Health Cooperative of Puget Sound [1]	WA	78

Better ⟵ ◐ ◑ ○ ◒ ● ⟶ Worse

Payment method for doctors. F indicates most primary-care doctors are paid fees for services; **C** indicates they receive a capitation payment; **S** means they receive a salary. **M** means any of the three methods is used.

Place of care. An **O** indicates predominant place of care is a physician's private office. **HC** means care is provided in a health center. Some HMOs provide care in both places. Those HMOs are indicated with an **O** and **HC**.

Family premiums. For HMOs that accept members who are not part of employer groups. HMOs not offering coverage to families are marked with a dash.

Medicare contract. Contract, if any, HMO has with the Health Care Financing Administration (HCFA) to provide Medicare benefits for members over 65. **Risk** contracts **(R)**, **cost** contracts **(C)**, and health-care prepayment plans, abbreviated here as **H**, are explained in greater detail in this chapter. A dash notes that plan does not contract with HCFA.

Medicare monthly premiums. Premiums that HMOs charge older members. Medicare plan may not be available in all locations.

Comments. Some benefits these HMOs offer and other dimensions of satisfaction, as rated by our respondents.

| | | Satisfaction with: | | | | | | | Medicare monthly premiums | |
HMO physician	Medical specialists	HMO administration	Payment method for doctors	Place of care	Family premiums	Medicare contract	Risk	Cost	Health care prepayment plan	Comments
◑	◑	◑	F	O	—	H	—	—	$66[3]	C,F,J,N,R,V
◑	◑	◉	F	O	—	—	—	—	—	B,E,I,M,Q,T,V
○	◑	◑	F	O	—	—	—	—	—	C,F,J,M,R
○	◑	◑	F	O	—	R	$87	—	—	D,E,H,M,Q
○	◑	○	F	O	—	R	85	—	—	D,E,K,M,Q
◑	◑	○	F	O	—	R	89[2][3]	—	—	[1],T,V
○	◉	○	F	O	$554[2]	H	—	—	93[2]	C,E,I,M,Q
◑	○	○	F,C	O	419	R	71[2]	—	—	C,E,J,M,Q,T,V
○	○	○	F,C	O,HC	427[3]	R	70	—	—	D,E,I,M,Q
○	○	◑	S	HC	449	R	38	—	—	B,E,I,M,P
○	○	○	S	HC,O	454[2]	R	107[2][3]	—	—	[1]

HMO	Service area	Satisfaction index
Columbia-Free State Health System	MD	78
Kaiser Foundation Health Plan	HI	78
HealthWays (now AETNA Healthplans of N.J./N.Y.)	NJ, Eastern PA	77
Harvard Community Health Plan	MA, NH, RI	77
MedCenters Health Plan [1]	MN, WI	77
HMO of Pennsylvania	PA, NJ	77
Kaiser Foundation Health Plan	Northern CA	77
Foundation Health Plan	Northern CA	76
Lifeguard [1]	CA	76
Share (now Medica Primary)	MN	76
Kaiser Foundation Health Plan	OR, WA	76
Kaiser Foundation Health Plan	Southern CA	75
Group Health Association (GHA)	DC, Northern VA, MD	75
Intergroup	AZ	75
Kaiser Foundation Health Plan	CO	75
TakeCare	CA	75
MD Individual Practice Association (MD-IPA)	MD, Northern VA, DC	75
AV-MED Health Plan	FL	74
FHP [1]	Southern CA	74
Kaiser Foundation Health Plan	OH	74
Kaiser Foundation Health Plan	DC, MD, Northern VA	73
HealthAmerica Corp. of Central Pennsylvania	PA	73
U.S. Healthcare (HMO of New Jersey)	NJ, Eastern PA	73
HMO Illinois [1]	IL	72
Compcare Health Services	WI	72
Health Net [1]	CA	72
Rush-Presbyterian St. Luke's (now Rush Anchor and Rush Access)	IL, IN	71
PacifiCare [1]	CA	70
Empire Blue Cross Blue Shield HealthNet	NY	69

| | Satisfaction with: | | | | | | Medicare monthly premiums | | | |
HMO physician	Medical specialists	HMO administration	Payment method for doctors	Place of care	Family premiums	Medicare contract	Risk	Cost	Health care prepayment plan	Comments
○	○	○	C	O, HC	574[3]	—	—	—	—	A,E,I,M,Q
○	○	○	S	HC	288	R, H	56[3]	—	70[4]	D,E,J,M,Q
●	○	○	F	O	—	C	—	$66[2]	—	C,E,I,M,Q
○	○	○	S	HC, O	465[2]	R	97[3]	—	—	D,E,K,M,Q
○	○	○	M	O	559	H	—	—	69[2]	[1]
○	○	○	C	O	—	R	55[2]	—	—	B,C,E,H,M,Q
○	○	○	S	HC	327[2]	H	—	—	61	D,E,J,M,Q
○	○	○	F, C	O	—	—	—	—	—	D,G,K,M,S,V
○	○	○	F	O	—	—	—	—	—	[1],V
○	●	○	C	O	—	R, C, H	52[2]	59	63	C,E,I,M,Q
○	○	○	S	HC	313	R, C	74[3]	63[4]	—	A,E,J,M,Q
○	○	○	S	HC	362	R, H	31	—	58[4]	D,E,J,M,Q
○	○	○	S	HC	414	H	—	—	99	C,E,I,M,Q
○	○	○	S, F	O	—	R	0	—	—	D,E,K,M,S
○	○	○	S	HC	324	R, H	62	—	51[4]	D,E,J,M,Q
○	○	○	M	O	—	—	—	—	—	D,E,J,M,R
○	○	○	C	O	—	—	—	—	—	D,E,K,M,Q
○	○	○	C	O	—	R	19	—	—	C,G,I,N,R
○	○	○	C, S	O, HC	419[2]	R	0	—	—	[1]
○	○	○	S	HC	377	R, H	62[3]	—	67[4]	D,E,J,M,Q
○	○	○	S	HC	386[2]	H	—	—	66[2]	D,E,J,M,Q
○	○	○	C	O	—	—	—	—	—	D,G,J,M,Q
○	○	○	C	O	—	—	—	—	—	B,C,E,H,M,Q
○	○	○	M	O	—	—	—	—	—	[1]
○	●	○	C	O	—	—	—	—	—	D,F,J,M,Q
○	○	○	M	O	—	—	—	—	—	[1]
○	○	◐	S, C	HC, O	—	C	—	66[2][3]	—	A,E,H,M,Q
○	○	○	[1]	[1]	—	R	10[2]	—	—	[1],U
○	○	○	F	O	—	—	—	—	—	D,E,J,M,Q

HMO	Service area	Satisfaction index
CIGNA Healthplans	Southern CA	68
Health Insurance Plan of Greater N.Y. (HIP)	NY	68
Michael Reese Health Plan (now Humana Michael Reese) 1	IL	67
Humana Medical Plan—South Florida	Southern FL	66
Sanus/New York Life Health Plan 1	Houston	65
CaliforniaCare	CA	63

1 Did not respond to a survey sent to HMO management.
2 May cost less in another location, or with fewer benefits, or for lower ages.

Key to Comments

A–Routine dental part of benefit plan.
B–Routine dental only for children.
C–Routine dental covered depending on the benefit plan, may cost more.
D–Routine dental not covered.
E–Routine eye exams for all ages covered.
F–Routine eye exams for all ages covered depending on the benefit plan, may cost more.
G–Routine eye exams for all ages not covered.
H–Eyeglasses covered as part of benefit plan.
I–Eyeglasses available from discounters.
J–Eyeglasses covered depending on the benefit plan, may cost more.
K–Eyeglasses not covered.
L–No limits on outpatient psychology visits.
M–Limited outpatient psychology visits.

98

| | Satisfaction with: | | | | | | | | Medicare monthly premiums | |
HMO physician	Medical specialists	HMO administration	Payment method for doctors	Place of care	Family premiums	Medicare contract	Risk	Cost	Health care prepayment plan	Comments
◑	◑	◑	S, C	HC, O	—	H	—	—	79[4]	D,E,N,S,U,W
◑	○	◑	S	HC	289[2]	R, H	35[2]	—	49[2][4]	D,E,J,M,Q,U,W
○	○	◑	S	HC	—	R	39[2]	—	[1]	,W
◑	◑	◑	C	O	—	R	0	—	—	C,F,J,N,R,U
◑	●	●	C	O	—	H	—	—	75	C,F,J,M,Q,U,W
●	●	●	S	O	610[2]	—	—	—	—	D,E,J,L,P,U,W

[3] *Only available during a specified enrollment period.*
[4] *Not currently open for new enrollment.*

N–Outpatient psychology covered depending on the benefit plan, may cost more.
O–Outpatient psychology not covered.
P–No limits on outpatient drug counseling.
Q–Limited number of outpatient drug counseling visits.
R–Outpatient drug counseling covered depending on the benefit plan, may cost more.
S–Outpatient drug counseling not covered.

T–Rated above average by members for thoroughness of exams.
U–Rated below average by members for thoroughness of exams.
V–Rated above average for times when appointments were available.
W–Rated below average for times when appointments were available.

the year if the HMO makes money. Those doctors have few incentives to overtreat, a problem that, as we saw in Chapter 1, plagues the U.S. health care system.

Others give primary-care doctors a "capitation" payment based on the number of patients who sign up for them. That payment is calculated to cover the expected cost of treating those patients over a given period. Doctors must make sure that the costs of care

---

"HMOs have developed ways to penalize doctors who send too many patients to hospitals or specialists."

---

do not exceed their capitation payments, because the doctors will receive no more money if they do. While a capitation payment eliminates incentives to overtreat, it can create incentives to undertreat. Since each visit takes up the doctor's time, and the doctor will receive no more money, he or she may discourage patients from seeking care for apparently trivial complaints that later turn out to be serious.

Other HMOs pay primary-care doctors fees for each service they perform. The HMO devises a fee schedule and pays accordingly. In most HMOs, specialists are also paid fees for their services, usually according to a fee schedule.

HMOs have developed ways to penalize doctors who send too many patients to hospitals or specialists. They may withhold a certain amount, usually 15 to 20 percent, of a doctor's capitation payment or of

each fee, in the case of physicians paid on a fee-for-service basis. At the end of the year, doctors get that money back only if the number of referrals and hospitalizations have not exceeded the HMO's targets.

Consumer Reports found a significant relationship between member satisfaction and the way primary-care doctors in the HMOs were paid. The HMOs at the top of our Ratings all paid doctors fees for their services.

Whatever method they use, most HMOs do not scrimp on payments to doctors and are mindful of what physicians can earn outside an HMO. If an HMO is not competitive in what it pays, doctors will drop out. "We spend an awful lot of time finding out what the marketplace is paying," says William McCoy, director of market development for Humana. "We want to be fair."

Because of those marketplace pressures, whatever increases doctors in traditional fee-for-service practices build into their fees each year eventually are reflected in what an HMO pays its doctors. That, obviously, undercuts the HMO's role as a controller of medical costs.

SEEING A SPECIALIST

Since HMO doctors may have a financial incentive to limit your access to specialists, it's not unreasonable to fear that you will be unable to see one. However, only 3 percent of our survey respondents complained that they could not see a specialist. Many more (14 percent) were dissatisfied with the choice of specialists made available to them. Members in plans

that paid primary-care doctors fees for their services were generally more satisfied with their specialists.

Physicians Health Plan of Minnesota, now called Medica Choice, received the highest rating for member satisfaction with specialists. That's not surprising, since that group's members can go to any specialist any time without obtaining a referral from a primary-care physician. On the other hand, at Sanus/New York Life Health Plan, which ranked near the bottom of our Ratings, 31 percent of our respondents were unhappy. That dissatisfaction may well be linked to the heavy penalty Sanus doctors pay if they refer too much. Twenty-five percent of their capitation payment can be withheld.

HMOs also limit referrals in other ways. Some require primary-care doctors to obtain approval before sending patients to hospitals or to specialists. Others limit the number of visits patients can have once they are referred. At Preferred Care in Rochester, New York, patients referred to dermatologists, plastic surgeons, and podiatrists are limited to six visits. Those restrictions apparently have not bothered members of Preferred Care, which was a cut above most other HMOs when it came to satisfaction with specialists.

NEW BREEDS OF MANAGED CARE

In the last few years, sellers of managed-care programs have created new arrangements for employees who are reluctant to enroll in traditional HMOs. The

differences—some slight and some not so slight—
between these plans and HMOs can affect how
patients get care. So if your employer offers one or
more of these options, it's crucial to understand how
the plans work and what they will cost you.

PPOs, or *preferred-provider organizations*, are networks of doctors and hospitals that have agreed to
give the sponsoring organization discounts from their
usual charges. These doctors and hospitals may be
the same ones the sponsors use for their HMOs, or
they may be different. In the basic PPO, doctors may
not go through a stringent credentialing process.
"We don't look at each physician," says Roy Oliver,
national practice director for KPMG Peat Marwick, a
consulting firm that selects PPO networks for
employers. Oliver says that his firm does try to make
sure there are enough doctors where employees live.

PPOs usually do not exercise tight management
over medical care. They may require doctors to
obtain the plan's approval before sending patients to
the hospital, but they do not require members to
choose a primary-care physician. If you join a basic
PPO, you can go to any doctor in the network whenever you want. That loose control over medical services raises questions about the PPO's potential to
control costs.

As long as you use network doctors, your employer
may pay 80 or 90 percent of your medical bills and, in
some plans, 100 percent. But if you go outside the network, your employer may pay only 60 or 70 percent.

Gatekeeper PPOs also have networks of hospitals and
doctors who have agreed to give discounts. But in

these arrangements, the sponsoring organization may pay more attention to the quality of its doctors. It may also more tightly control the use of medical services, much the way an HMO does. You will have to choose a primary-care physician, as you would in an HMO. That doctor will be responsible for your care and will make all referrals to specialists. If you stay in the network, you will receive a higher benefit than if you go outside. If you go to doctors outside the PPO, you may have to pay as much as 40 percent of the bill, unless your primary-care doctor referred you to the outside physician.

A number of managed-care companies have taken their gatekeeper PPOs one step further. They have created plans that pay no benefits if members go outside the network. These plans, called *exclusive-provider organizations,* or EPOs, resemble HMOs but are usually regulated under state insurance laws, not the statutes governing HMOs. As a result, they may lack some consumer safeguards, such as quality-assurance programs and the formal grievance procedures found in real HMOs.

Opt-out or *point-of-service HMOs,* the latest fashion in managed care, are regular HMOs with one critical difference. When you go into a regular HMO, you get all your care from plan physicians and, in return, you pay either nominal copayments or nothing at all. If you go outside the HMO, you have to cover the entire cost yourself. But in an opt-out arrangement, your employer's plan will pay some of the cost, usually 60 or 70 percent, if you obtain care outside the HMO. The HMO's usual grievance procedures and quality-assurance programs will apply as long as you stay within the network. But if you go outside the network, you lose the HMO's oversight of the care you receive.

Specialized networks, designed for certain medical problems, such as mental illness or substance abuse, combine the network features of HMOs and PPOs with utilization-review tools. The objective of these networks is to cut inpatient hospital treatment for mental illness and substance abuse, which is costly and sometimes inappropriate. Employers who purchase services from these networks require employees to phone the network before seeking care. The sponsoring organization usually sends employees to health-care providers that offer the sponsor discounts.

As with PPOs and opt-out HMOs, employees can go outside the network for care. But if they do, their reimbursement will be smaller. Typically, employers' plans will pay 80 percent of the cost of treatment for employees who stay in the network and only 50 percent if they go outside.

QUESTIONS OF QUALITY

Ask any HMO or managed-care outfit about the quality of care it provides, and its answer will probably focus on how it chooses its doctors or what their offices look like, rather than on whether their doctors practice clinically appropriate medicine. Most plans have no scientific measures for determining the quality of health care for various conditions.

What instead passes for quality assurance in many

HMOs: DO THEY MEAN LONGER WAITS FOR CARE?

We asked respondents who belong to HMOs and respondents with traditional health insurance how long they had to wait for a doctor's appointment and how long they had to wait in the doctor's office. As the graph shows, HMO members had to wait a little longer for appointments, but once they got to the doctor's office, their waits were shorter, belying the image of HMOs as places where people wait hours for their care.

HMOs ━━━
Insurance ▪▪▪▪

Waits for nonemergency appointments

over 2 months	
over 1 month	
3-4 weeks	
1-2 weeks	
3-6 days	
1-2 days	

0   10%   20%   30%   40%   50%

Waits past the appointed time in doctors' offices

over 1 hour	
over 30 minutes	
15-30 minutes	
less than 15 minutes	

0   10%   20%   30%   40%   50%

BUT SOME HMOs WERE BETTER THAN OTHERS

Respondents rated the following HMOs better than average or worse than average for waiting times.

The shortest waits for appointments

AV-MED Health Plan
Comprecare
Foundation Health Plan
HealthWays (Aetna of N.J./N.Y.)
Heritage National Health Plan
HMO of Pennsylvania
MD Individual Practice Association (MD-IPA)
Sanus/New York Life Health Plan (Houston)
U.S. Healthcare (HMO of New Jersey)

The longest waits for appointments

Group Health Association (GHA)
Health Alliance Plan
Health Insurance Plan of Greater N.Y.
Kaiser (Colorado)
Kaiser (Mid-Atlantic)
Kaiser (Northern Calif.)
Kaiser (Northwest)
Kaiser (Ohio)
Kaiser (Southern Calif.)
Michael Reese Health Plan (Humana Michael Reese)

The shortest waits in doctors' offices

Columbia-Free State Health System
Comprecare
Group Health Association (GHA)
Group Health Cooperative of Puget Sound
Group Health, Inc.
Harvard Community Health Plan
Kaiser (Northern Calif.)
Kaiser (Northwest)
MedCenters Health Plan
Physicians Health Plan of Minnesota (Medica Choice)
Share (Medica Primary)

The longest waits in doctors' offices

CaliforniaCare
Empire Blue Cross Blue Shield (HealthNet)
Health Insurance Plan of Greater N.Y.
HealthWays (Aetna of N.J./N.Y.)
Humana Medical Plan (South Fla.)
Independent Health

HMOs are chart reviews in which the HMO determines whether the chart is legible and notes if a doctor has told patients to stop smoking or has checked their blood pressure. But simply totaling the number of doctors' offices that checked patients for hypertension hardly addresses how well doctors treated patients with the disease.

Some HMOs point to their consumer satisfaction surveys, which invariably show that members are happy with the plan and, by implication, with the quality of care they received. But what a member thinks is high-quality care may not be that at all. When HMOs themselves have seriously investigated quality, they have found it wanting.

In the area of preventive care, many HMOs have yet to fulfill their mission. Consider immunizations, for example. Immunization rates for children have been falling across the country, leaving children at

---

"In the area of preventive care, many HMOs have yet to fulfill their mission."

---

risk for such easily preventable diseases as measles and diphtheria. HMOs could lead the medical community by making sure that all their young members have been immunized, but they have not done so. Although immunizations are free to HMO members, and HMOs could easily remind members when it's time to come in for shots, immunization rates at HMOs range only from 60 to 85 percent.

If quality of care is difficult to measure, quality of

service is not. Delays in getting through on the telephone, waits for appointments or in doctors' offices, the doctor's "bedside manner," and the plan's responsiveness to questions and complaints all affect a member's happiness with an HMO. Generally, the top-rated HMOs in our survey scored well on those dimensions, and the ones at the bottom fared relatively poorly. Overall, nearly half of those we surveyed waited at least one week to get an appointment for nonemergency care. But at HMOs rated above average, less than 25 percent experienced such waits.

Members who receive their care in health centers generally had to wait longer for appointments than those who receive care in doctors' offices. Most Kaiser plans, where members get their care at centers, were worse than average. At HIP in New York, 70 percent of the members waited at least a week.

THE 'UTILIZATION REVIEW' PROCESS

At her workstation in a modern office building near Philadelphia, Maureen Thomas, R.N., takes a call from the wife of a 74-year-old man who has just been admitted to a local emergency room with a blood clot in his leg. The man's insurance policy requires him to notify Thomas's employer, Intracorp, whenever he goes to the hospital.

The man is too ill to phone, so his wife has done it for him. Nurse Thomas types information about his condition into her computer and tells his wife he will initially be assigned a hospital stay of only one day.

Later that afternoon, when she knows more about the prognosis, Thomas authorizes a four-day stay, which her computer says is appropriate for a person with his condition. After four days he must either go home or Thomas and the man's doctor will have to agree on additional days of hospitalization. If the patient stays without permission from Intracorp, he may have to pay for the unauthorized hospital days himself.

Welcome to the world of managed care as it's now being practiced by insurance companies attempting to control health-care costs. Policies that once allowed medical decisions to be made by you and your doctor now call for intervention by nurses like Thomas who work for *utilization review* firms, which number around 260 across the nation.

A number of different services fall under the rubric of utilization review: the "hospital preauthorization" that Nurse Thomas was performing; "second opinion reviews," in which the firm decides whether a second opinion for a surgical procedure is necessary; "prospective procedure review," in which a nurse says you can have certain surgeries or diagnostic tests if your condition meets specific criteria; "concurrent review," in which a nurse continuously reviews your charts while you are in the hospital; and "case management," in which a manager coordinates your care and rehabilitation, often at your home.

Utilization-review companies aggressively sell their services to employers and to other insurance companies. (Some are themselves owned by big health insurers.) HMOs and preferred-provider organizations use them, too. Some utilization-review firms specialize in particular illnesses, such as mental-health problems. At least one handles only foot care.

For a monthly fee of $1 to $3 per patient, the firms propose to cut the number of days employees spend in hospitals or the number of surgical operations performed on them. And, as a result, the firms promise to save their customers big money. Saving that big money has become a big business. In 1991, utilization-review companies grossed an estimated $7.4 billion. Intracorp alone employs 2,400 nurses to pass judgment on some 800,000 hospital admissions each year.

Utilization review has prevented some unnecessary surgery, kept some people out of hospitals, and steered others to more appropriate care. And in doing so it has probably saved some employers some money. But accounting for *how much* money has stirred debate, since there's no uniform way to collect data or measure the results. Furthermore, some utilization-review firms overstate the savings they report.

To measure the savings, firms typically compare the number of days a doctor requests for a hospital stay with the number of days the firms actually approve. They then multiply the difference by the cost of a day in the hospital to arrive at a total savings figure that they report to employers. But estimating savings this way does not take into account that doctors may routinely request more days than they expect to need for a given patient, just to be on the safe side in case of a complication. For example, a surgeon whose gallbladder patients stay an average of four days may request six days, knowing that the review firm will approve only four. When that happens, the two extra days are reported as savings, though the patient would have stayed only four days anyway.

Firms that specialize in mental health also report big savings, but possibly at the expense of patient care. Some mental health review firms claim that in the first year they can cut by half the amount an employer spends on psychiatric and substance-abuse treatment for its workers. However, David Noone, president of Preferred Health Care, a large mental health review firm, says a 20- or 30-percent cut is more realistic. "You don't want 50-percent savings," he said. "They are probably denying care."

CONTAINING COSTS?

We asked the HMOs in our study to rank various utilization-review tools in terms of their effectiveness at cutting the use of medical services and, therefore, the costs. There was no consensus. Where one HMO thought that prescreening hospital admissions was very valuable, another said it was not. Insurance carriers and utilization-review firms do not agree, either. Aetna, an insurer, offers a service called "managed second opinion": Policyholders contemplating, say, gallbladder surgery have to phone for permission to have the operation; if Aetna considers the person a poor candidate for the procedure, it reviews the case again and sometimes asks for another exam. Intracorp, by contrast, once required policyholders to phone for permission to have gallbladder surgery but found that doing so did not reduce the number of operations that were done. So it dropped gallbladder surgery and 25 other procedures from its review list. Now policyholders must seek approval for only seven procedures and diagnostic tests.

If the cost savings that result from utilization review are hard to quantify, the administrative burdens imposed by it and other managed-care programs are not. Administrative expenses for the managed-care programs are 10 to 18 percent of the premiums collected, compared with 4 to 12 percent for traditional insurance products.

The process also increases administrative burdens on physicians, who may have to deal with several review firms each week. Some firms may call daily to inquire about patients they want out of the hospital. "Every firm is looking for something different," says a former nurse reviewer for John Hancock who did not want to be identified. "It's an administrative nightmare for doctors to keep the various protocols for each one correct."

Utilization review comes at a cost to patients as well. There's no uniformity among the review firms in how they apply the tools of their trade. The kind of treatment you can expect may vary from firm to firm and will even depend on the orders your employer has given the company. "We don't have one standard approach," says Ronald Gomes, an Intracorp vice president. If an employer instructs the firm to take a soft approach, the nurse may be more lenient in allowing someone to go to the hospital. If the employer says to take a harder line, the nurse may be quicker to say "no."

The utilization-review industry is largely unregulated, with few outside standards for review criteria or protocols. In most states, firms need not reveal how they do their reviews. Secrecy is necessary, they say, to keep doctors from getting around the rules. But the patient can be caught in the middle, denied treatment and unable to learn why. "All of us have horror stories about clients who were left in states of dysfunction because their treatment had to be prematurely terminated," a social worker in Albany, New York, told *Consumer Reports*.

Only one thing is really certain in the brave new world of managed care: It puts additional burdens on sick people to remember their plan's requirements. If you arrive in acute pain at the emergency room, you had better be sure you, your spouse, or your next-door neighbor knows the rules of your insurance plan, or you could lose your benefits for "noncompliance."

WHAT YOU PAY

HMO members usually receive more benefits for their premiums than patients with traditional insurance do. Those benefits can include preventive care, such as annual physicals, immunizations, and well-baby visits. Plans may also provide eyeglasses, prescription drugs, and dental treatment, sometimes for an extra premium. Our Ratings show some of the benefits the plans offer.

The Health Insurance Association of America found that monthly premiums for family coverage in

1990 averaged $311 for HMOs that provided care mainly through health centers and $316 for those that provided care in physicians' offices. Monthly premiums for health insurance with managed-care features averaged $319.

Even though there may be little difference in premiums between HMOs and traditional insurance, HMOs have had an edge when it comes to copayments and deductibles. Copayments for office visits have historically been small ($2 was common) compared with the 20 percent of the doctor's fee required by traditional insurance. Deductibles usually were nonexistent, but that's changing now, as employers shift the burden of their increasing health costs to their workers.

Employees enrolled in HMOs are facing higher copayments and, in some HMOs, deductibles. Copayments now run from $5 to $10 per office visit and from $25 to $500 per hospital admission. Still, with an HMO, your out-of-pocket costs are likely to be lower and more predictable. Survey respondents in HMOs whose premiums were not totally covered by

---

"Deductibles usually were nonexistent, but that's changing now, as employers shift the burden of increasing health costs to their workers."

---

their employers typically paid about $60 a month for their share of the costs, while those with traditional coverage paid $80.

Seventy-two percent of our respondents in HMOs who needed hospital treatment reported that their plans covered their total hospital bills. Those who had to pay out-of-pocket expenses averaged only $100. In contrast, only 40 percent of our respondents who had traditional insurance said the carriers covered their hospital bills in full. For those who had to pay, out-of-pocket expenses averaged $500.

If you are not in a group health plan and need to buy individual coverage, you may do better at an HMO than with an insurance company. At Comprecare in Denver, family coverage for a man of 40, a wife of 40, and two children runs about $419 a month; at Kaiser of Colorado, such coverage would cost about $325. The Comprecare plan requires copayments of $10 for office visits and $100 for each hospital admission. Kaiser's plan requires a $10 copayment for both. In comparison, the same family would pay $442 a month for a good policy from American Republic, one of the top-rated insurers in our 1990 study of health insurance. That policy requires no coinsurance but has a deductible of $750. If the family increased the deductible to $1,000, they'd pay $395 a month.

However, if you are not part of a group, you may have trouble finding an HMO that will take you. Only 22 percent of all HMOs cover people under age 65 who are not part of employer groups. If you are able to find an HMO that takes individuals, you will have to meet its medical requirements. HMOs, like insurance companies, want people who are healthy, so if you recently had cancer or are a diabetic, forget about getting individual coverage. If an HMO does accept you, though, there will often be no waiting period for coverage for pre-existing health conditions and no permanent exclusions for any medical problem you already have. What's more, your benefits will be as good as everyone else's.

The Ratings chart in this chapter shows which plans accept individuals under 65 who are not part of a group.

CONSIDERING HMO COVERAGE

If you work for a large employer that offers an HMO, you can sign up for a plan no matter what your health status. If you work for a small employer, your health, the health of your colleagues, and the number of people who enroll all count.

HMOs are somewhat more lenient than insurance companies when it comes to insuring small groups. They will either offer coverage to everyone or reject the entire group. If some employees in the group have chronic conditions that are likely to raise costs, the HMO may simply say "no" to all, not take some employees and reject others, the way insurance companies do. An HMO may also reject a group if too few employees sign up, or if the group is part of a "problem" industry that is likely to generate claims. Comprecare, a high-rated HMO, avoids insuring people who work in hospitals. "People who work in hospitals are exposed to the newest technology and drugs," says an underwriter for the HMO. "They know what they want and tend to use the highest priced services."

If you leave your job, most likely you can remain on your employer's plan and retain your HMO

117

benefits, usually for 18 months. After that, you will have to find other insurance or convert to individual coverage within the HMO. Most HMOs offer such conversions. Generally, conversion coverage at an HMO will provide better benefits than a conversion policy an insurance company might offer you. With the exception of prescription drugs, the benefits for HMO coverage will usually be the same ones you received as a part of a group.

Many HMOs will let you continue your coverage for the same premium or for one slightly higher than you were paying for group coverage. At Pilgrim Health Care, for example, a group premium for a single person in Norwell, Massachusetts, comes to about $2,130 a year. Comparable conversion coverage comes to $2,328. With a health insurance company, a person converting from group coverage to an individual policy might pay thousands of dollars more for far fewer benefits.

If you are in your 50s and concerned that you might lose your job and then have no coverage except for a conversion policy, consider joining an HMO now. If you are later forced to take a conversion, you will get a better deal from most HMOs than from insurance companies.

Some HMOs offer plans to replace regular Medicare and Medigap coverage (see Chapter 4).

THE ISSUE OF STABILITY

As employers search for cheaper premiums, and as HMOs themselves change their networks to control costs and improve medical care, members may find themselves buffeted from HMO to HMO or to some other kind of managed-care plan. The *Consumer Reports* survey shows that the major reason people have left their HMOs in the past three years is simply that the plans were no longer offered to them.

During the 1980s, many entrepreneurs rushed to start HMOs. Some HMOs ran into financial trouble when medical costs climbed in the 1980s. As a result, many HMOs have been bought, sold, merged, or shut down altogether. (One highly rated HMO in our study, Bay State Health Care, encountered financial problems a few years ago; Blue Cross/Blue Shield of Massachusetts recently took it over.) If your HMO changes hands or goes out of business and your coverage is picked up by another plan, your benefits may not be exactly the same. Whether you lose coverage altogether depends on state laws and on whether your employer offers other insurance options.

RATING SERVICES AND COSTS

Many employed people today have the choice of an HMO, another managed-care plan such as a preferred-provider organization, or an old-fashioned insurance policy with some newfangled managed-care features. If you work for a large employer, you may even have a choice among HMOs.

To find out how HMOs stacked up against traditional insurance and against each other, we asked *Consumer Reports* readers who belonged to an HMO to rate their medical experiences from spring 1990 through spring 1991. We also asked readers with traditional coverage to rate similar medical experiences over the same period. (Our respondents in both surveys were relatively healthy.)

Respondents in HMOs were just as satisfied as those with ordinary coverage. We found no meaningful differences in such factors as the number of office visits they had, the length of the typical visit, the ability to get answers to questions by telephone, the number of specialists seen, or the waiting times to see a specialist. We also found that members in HMOs and those with traditional insurance were equally satisfied with the way medical personnel explained diagnoses and treatments, their willingness to listen to questions, availability of doctors and labs for appointments, and the thoroughness of exams.

When it came to satisfaction with out-of-pocket costs, HMO members were far happier than those with traditional insurance. That's the result of a trade-off, of course. When you join an HMO, you lose much of the freedom to go to any doctor you want. But the combination of lower out-of-pocket costs and coverage for preventive services may make it a good choice for many people.

CAN HMOS CONTROL COSTS?

The HMOs in our survey generally satisfied their members at least as well as traditional fee-for-service practitioners, and some do a good job of holding down the out-of-pocket costs for individual members. For those reasons, you may wish to join one. But when it comes to holding down the nation's $800-billion medical bill, the story of HMOs is less clear-cut.

As already noted, our respondents were largely satisfied with HMOs. They went to the doctor as often as those who had traditional insurance, saw the same number of specialists, and were almost never denied medical tests they thought they should have. In other words, they appeared to use as many medical services as people outside an HMO do.

HMO members were a little less likely to go to the hospital for an overnight stay, and, when they did go, they stayed one day less on average. "Hospital use tends to be lower in HMOs, but there's a wide range from plan to plan in how much lower," says Dr. Harold Luft, professor of health economics at the University of California, San Francisco. "Ambulatory care [given to patients outside of hospitals] is not lower and, if anything, may be higher in the HMO."

Academic studies have suggested that prepaid group health plans, in which members received the bulk of their care in health centers, delivered medical services at a lower cost than traditional arrangements. Most of the cost reductions were achieved by negotiating discounts with hospitals and by reducing the number of days members spent in them. HMOs also tended to attract younger, healthier people, which may have affected the amount spent on medical care.

HMOs still draw a younger crowd, but the number of days the U.S. population as a whole stays in the hospital has come down substantially since the late 1970s; thus, any further savings to the HMO in that area are likely to be less dramatic. And the provider discounts—whether from hospitals, drug companies, or doctors—have simply caused providers to shift higher costs to other users of their services. A hospital that agrees to lower its prices for an HMO may simply raise them to others. Thus a cost shifted by an HMO is not a cost saved for the nation.

Furthermore, the fastest-growing HMOs are those in which doctors practice in their own offices and often get paid per service, rather than those with health centers and salaried doctors, where controls may be tighter. In fee-for-service HMOs, there's pressure to pay physicians fees that are close to those charged by doctors in traditional practices outside the HMO.

HMOs cannot easily control the costliest doctors in their networks—that is, the specialists and superspecialists. Anesthesiologists, pathologists, and emergency-room physicians are difficult to bring into a network at all.

Finally, pressure to use expensive, new technology is as pervasive inside the HMO as it is outside. The case of Preferred Care is instructive. In 1992, Preferred Care, one of our top-rated HMOs and one that pays doctors a fee for each service they perform, increased payments to doctors by 17 percent. Half the increase directly boosted doctors' fees; the other half covered the cost of the growing number of medical services. The HMO found, for example, that its radiologists were performing more, costlier procedures, such as magnetic resonance imaging, which lets doctors see tissues inside the body without radiation.

"We're not proud we've had these big rate increases," says Leon Gossin, Preferred Care's manager of financial planning. "HMOs have done better than indemnity insurers [at controlling costs], but not as well as they should have."

ADVICE TO CONSUMERS: CHOOSING MANAGED CARE

Periodically, typically in the fall, your employer may offer an open-enrollment period during which you can change your health insurance coverage. If so, you may face a bewildering choice of managed-care plans.

If a plan you are considering is not in our Ratings, you may have little to go on beyond the advice of your employee-benefits manager. And even then, your company may have chosen an HMO or other managed-care plan not because it offers quality service and quality medical care but because it gave the employer an exceptionally good price.

Besides looking at such obvious points as cost and coverage, there are other important things to keep in mind. Here's a list of questions to ask:

- When must I notify the plan before going to the hospital or in the case of an emergency, and how do I do it? Some managed-care plans require you to obtain approval before going to a hospital; in others, such as HMOs and preferred-provider organizations (PPOs), your doctor usually obtains permission for you. If you ignore the rules, you could jeopardize your benefits.

- Will I be penalized for going outside the network? Your share of the costs can vary, depending on whether you choose an HMO, a PPO, or an opt-out HMO. But just knowing the cost-sharing amounts is not enough. You need to know how they are applied. If your plan covers 80 percent of the cost, does that 80 percent apply to the doctor's actual charge or to what the plan determines is an allowable charge? If the doctor charges $8,000, but the plan allows only $3,000 for a procedure, you would receive only $2,400 (80 percent of $3,000). You would still owe the doctor $5,600.

- What happens if I see a specialist who is not in the plan? That may happen if you belong to a PPO. If your primary-care doctor refers you, you usually will get the higher "in-network" benefits. If you choose the specialist yourself, you may get lower benefits.

- Are all services offered by a doctor in a network covered? A plan may authorize a doctor, for example, to perform routine gynecology, but not infertility treatment.

- Who pays if my regular doctor is unavailable and another doctor is covering? Will the covering physician be able to collect from the managed-care plan, or will he or she bill me for payment?

- Is there a doctor nearby? HMOs and PPOs provide directories for members to use in choosing physicians. But before you sign up, make sure the plan has enough primary-care doctors and specialists in your area.

- Are doctors in the plan taking any new patients? Look skeptically at plans whose directories indicate that many of the listed doctors are not: The HMO or PPO organization may be keeping those doctors in its directory simply to make the book look fatter, or the doctors may be dissatisfied with the plan and not want to accept any new patients from among its members.

- Are the doctors who belong to the plan board-certified, meaning that they have passed certain tests for competency in their medical field? Have they been with the plan long? Are there grievances or complaints against them? The HMO or PPO may be reluctant to tell you, so be persistent.

- How is the doctor paid? Readers generally liked plans that paid primary-care doctors fees for their services.

- Is the doctor I'm considering satisfied with the plan? Call and ask. If a doctor is unhappy, either because he or she is not paid in a timely way or for other reasons, you probably want to pick another doctor—or another plan for that matter. A dissatisfied doctor may be on the verge of dropping out, which would disrupt your care.

- What is the doctor's obligation to me if he or she leaves the plan while I'm in the hospital? The plan may require the doctor to continue your treatment until you are discharged.

- If my employer asks me to switch plans during the course of treatment or during a pregnancy, can I stay with my current physician until the treatment or the pregnancy is completed? Some plans will allow you to do that, others will not.

- How does the plan handle mental-health coverage? What are the benefits? Who determines the care I will receive—the organization itself or a utilization-review company it hires? What recourse do I have if I'm unhappy with my care?

4
HEALTH COVERAGE FOR THOSE 65 AND OVER

"Medigap policies have proliferated, and so have marketing abuses."

S ince its creation in 1965, the federal government's Medicare program has provided a substantial safety net to older Americans. For relatively healthy people whose doctors charge modest fees, and who do not need costly prescription drugs, Medicare still comes close to meeting its original mandate to protect people over 65 from burdensome health care expenditures.

But from the beginning, Medicare has also contained coverage gaps that, for some, can cause real financial hardship. Hospital deductibles, copayments, and the cost of prescription drugs can add up rapidly for people with serious or chronic illnesses.

Today, Medicare beneficiaries face out-of-pocket costs that border on being unaffordable. For the first 60 days of hospital care, for instance, beneficiaries must pay a deductible of $652; Medicare pays the rest of the bill through its Part A coverage, which takes care of hospital services. For the 61st through 90th days, beneficiaries must pay $163 per day towards their hospital bill. Obviously, most people do not stay in the hospital nearly that long, but those who do can see their bills consume a lifetime's savings in a matter of weeks.

Similarly, Medicare pays only 80 percent of physicians' allowed charges under its Part B section, which covers medical services. Beneficiaries must pay the other 20 percent. Allowed charges used to be derived from the average fees charged by doctors in a particular area. But beginning in 1992, allowed charges are determined by the level of skill and the time required to do a particular procedure, modified by geographic factors such as the cost of office rents and the prevailing salaries for office help. That means, for instance, that a doctor in New York City is likely to be allowed to charge more for a given procedure than a doctor in, say, rural Kansas.

Doctors who do not accept the Medicare-allowed charge as full payment are permitted to bill as much as 20 percent above the Medicare fee level; beneficiaries are responsible for this extra charge as well. Finally, with a few minor exceptions, Medicare does not include any coverage for prescription drugs taken outside the hospital.

To fill these gaps in coverage, private insurance to supplement Medicare, popularly known as "Medigap" policies, has existed alongside Medicare from its earliest days. In the early days of Medicare, when health care costs were much lower than they are now, out-of-pocket expenses were lower as well. So were Medigap premiums. As health care costs began their historical climb, so did the out-of-pocket payments and premiums. Along the way, Medigap policies have proliferated, and so have marketing abuses. A 1989 investigation by *Consumer Reports* uncovered numerous problems in the design and marketing of Medigap policies. Too often, sales agents were peddling inadequate or duplicative plans using misleading information.

To bring some order to this market, in 1990 Congress passed legislation mandating the creation of 10 standardized Medigap policies. The legislation gave the job of actually designing the policies to the National Association of Insurance Commissioners (NAIC), which writes model legislation for states to adopt.

The policies began appearing in 1992, as states adopted the NAIC packages, designated by the letters A through J. Medigap insurers will be able to sell only those policies. They all must offer the most basic package, Plan A; they do not have to offer the others. While each standardized plan will be identical from insurer to insurer, prices may differ. Not all policies may be available in all states. Three states—Massachusetts, Minnesota, and Wisconsin—had already standardized their Medigap policies and were grandfathered out of the new regulations. In these states, companies must offer a core policy plus standardized optional riders.

MEDIGAP COVERAGE

All 10 plans include certain core benefits. Plan A offers only these benefits, and no others. The plans are examined in more detail in the following pages.

The core benefit plan does not include the $652 deductible that beneficiaries must pay for the first 60 days of a hospital stay. But the plan does cover the $163-a-day copayment imposed for days 61 through 90, and the $326-a-day copayment imposed for days 91 through 150. For truly catastrophic hospital stays of longer than 150 days, the core plan includes total coverage for another 365 days of care. The core plan also covers the so-called Part A blood deductible, under which the patient is responsible for the first three pints of blood administered during a hospital stay.

As for doctor bills, the core plan pays the recipient's 20 percent share of the doctor's allowable charge. The core benefits also include total coverage for another 365 days of care after all other Medicare hospital benefits are exhausted.

The core plan does not cover some potentially costly out-of-pocket liabilities, however. Medicare, for instance, will cover in full only the first 20 days in a skilled-nursing facility, and even then under strictly limited conditions: The patient must come to the nursing home straight from a hospital stay of at least three days and be certified by a doctor as needing skilled care. For days 21 through 100, Medicare recipients must pay $81.50 a day towards their bill. The core plan does not cover this copayment.

The core plan also will not pay for physicians' "excess charges," which are bills that exceed Medicare's allowable charge. As noted above, beginning this year, nonparticipating doctors cannot charge more than 20 percent above the allowable schedule; in 1993, the excess charge can be no more than 15 percent of the allowable charge. Even though doctors can no longer charge Medicare patients fees as large as they wish to, Consumers Union still believes that coverage for excess charges is a good idea.

All policies, except Plans A and B, cover emergency medical treatment in foreign countries, and all except Plan A pay the Part A deductible, this year $652. Only three policies pay the $100 Part B deductible, and fewer than half cover care needed at home following a hospital stay for an acute illness. The at-home recovery benefit pays for assistance with "activities of daily living," such as eating, bathing, and dressing, provided that the insured person also qualifies for Medicare home-care benefits. That benefit is not a substitute for coverage offered by long-term care insurance policies.

Two policies cover preventive medical care, which includes hearing tests, flu vaccines, and tests for thyroid function, diabetes, and colo-rectal cancer. Three pay for prescription drugs, up to a maximum of $1,250 or $3,000, depending on the plan. Policyholders who buy those plans must still pay the first $250 of their annual drug bills, as well as half the cost of each prescription.

THE 10 STANDARDIZED PLANS

In 1990, Congress delegated the NAIC to create 10 standardized Medicare-supplement policies. Companies can now offer *only* the 10 prescribed plans. Each plan is the same from insurer to insurer: One company's Plan C is identical to another's Plan C. Therefore, the main differences among policies are price and the quality of the service provided by the insurance company.

Not all 10 policies may be approved for sale in your state, however, and not every insurance company offers every plan. Once you decide which plan suits your needs, seek out the companies that sell that particular plan. If the plan of your choice is not offered in your state (your state insurance department can tell you this), then choose the one that is available and comes closest to meeting your requirements.

The following is a guide to the types of coverage provided by each Medicare-supplement plan.

Plan A. Every insurer must offer Plan A, which provides certain core, or basic, benefits. These include:

1. Coverage for Part A coinsurance—the daily amount you must pay for a hospital stay if

you are hospitalized from 61 to 90 days. In 1992, Part A coinsurance is $163 a day.

2. Coverage for Part A coinsurance—the daily amount you must pay for a hospital stay that lasts from 91 to 150 days. In 1992, that amount is $326.

3. Coverage for an extra 365 days of hospital care after you have exhausted all of your Medicare benefits. Insurance companies usually reimburse hospitals according to the prospective payment system that Medicare uses.

4. Coverage for the cost of the first three pints of blood you may need as an inpatient in a hospital. In other words, policies will cover the Part A blood deductible.

5. Coverage for Part B coinsurance—20 percent of Medicare's allowable charge.

Plan B. Plan B must include the core benefits, plus the following:

1. Coverage for coinsurance for a stay in a skilled-nursing facility. Medicare requires beneficiaries needing skilled-nursing care to pay coinsurance for stays that last from 21 to 100 days. In 1992, the amount of the coinsurance is $81.50. After that, neither Medicare nor Medicare-supplement insurance pays any part of the bill.

2. Part A hospital deductible. This is $652 in 1992.

133

Plan C. Plan C must include the core benefits, plus the following:
1. Coverage for coinsurance for a stay in a skilled-nursing facility.
2. Part A hospital deductible.
3. Emergency medical care in foreign countries.
4. Part B deductible—$100 in 1992.

Plan D. Plan D includes the core benefits, plus:
1. Coverage for coinsurance for a stay in a skilled-nursing facility.
2. Part A hospital deductible.
3. Emergency medical care in foreign countries.
4. Coverage for at-home care following an injury, illness, or surgery. This benefit covers assistance with activities of daily living such as eating, bathing, and dressing. *Note:* The at-home care coverage provided is limited to a short period. For example, the benefit is limited to $1,600 per year, and your physician must certify that visits by a licensed home-health aide or homemaker or personal-care worker are necessary because of a condition for which Medicare has already approved a home-health care treatment plan for you.

Plan E. Plan E includes the core benefits, plus the following:
1. Coverage for coinsurance for a stay in a

skilled-nursing facility.
2. Part A hospital deductible.
3. Emergency medical care in foreign countries.
4. Preventive medical care. This benefit covers the cost of an annual physical, fecal occult blood tests, mammograms, thyroid and diabetes screening, a pure-tone hearing test, and cholesterol screening every five years.

Plan F. Plan F contains the core benefits, plus the following:
1. Coverage for coinsurance for a stay in a skilled-nursing facility.
2. Part A hospital deductible.
3. Part B deductible.
4. Emergency medical care in foreign countries.
5. One hundred percent of Medicare Part B excess charges. An excess charge is the difference between Medicare's approved amount or allowed charge and the amount the physician actually bills.

Plan G. Plan G includes the core benefits, plus the following:
1. Coverage for coinsurance for a stay in a skilled-nursing facility.
2. Part A hospital deductible.
3. Emergency medical care in foreign countries.
4. Coverage for at-home care following an

injury, illness, or surgery.
5.   Eighty percent of Medicare Part B excess
     charges.

Plan H. Plan H includes the core benefits, plus the
following:
1.   Coverage for coinsurance for a stay in a
     skilled-nursing facility.
2.   Part A hospital deductible.
3. . Emergency medical care in foreign
     countries.
4.   Coverage for at-home care following an
     injury, illness, or surgery.
5.   Fifty percent of the cost of prescription
     drugs up to an annual maximum benefit of
     $1,250 after the policyholder satisfies a $250
     annual deductible. This is the basic prescrip-
     tion drug benefit.

Plan I. Plan I includes the core benefits, plus the
following:
1.   Coverage for coinsurance for a stay in a
     skilled-nursing facility.
2.   Part A hospital deductible.
3.   Emergency medical care in foreign
     countries.
4.   Coverage for at-home care following an
     injury, illness, or surgery.
5.   One hundred percent of Part B excess
     charges.
6.   The basic prescription drug benefit.

Plan J. Plan J includes the core benefits, plus the following:

1. Coverage for coinsurance for a stay in a skilled-nursing facility.
2. Part A hospital deductible.
3. Part B deductible.
4. Emergency medical care in foreign countries.
5. Coverage for at-home care following an injury, illness, or surgery.
6. Preventive medical care.
7. One hundred percent of Part B excess charges.
8. Fifty percent of the cost of prescription drugs up to an annual maximum benefit of $3,000 after the policyholder meets an annual $250 deductible. This is the extended drug benefit.

TRADEOFFS: PRICE VS. COVERAGE

The more coverage you want, the more you'll pay. Plan A, with only the most basic benefits, may cost as little as $300 or $400 a year, depending on where you live and your age when you buy the policy. Plan J, the most comprehensive, may cost as much as $2,000 a year.

What a company charges may also depend on how thoroughly it "underwrites"—that is, scrutinizes the health of prospective policyholders. A carrier that underwrites stringently may be able to charge less

because it accepts only the healthiest people. But note, however, that the new rules prohibit insurers from checking on the health of applicants age 65 and older during the first six months after they sign up for Medicare Part B. That means it's important for people with chronic health conditions (heart ailments, for instance) to buy a Medicare-supplement policy as soon as they sign up for Medicare. Once the six-month period is up, they may find they cannot buy insurance at any price because their health presents too much of a risk for the insurance carrier.

Companies that offer plans paying for prescription drugs are likely to check applicants' health carefully, and people who already use prescription drugs may have a hard time buying drug coverage.

If you already own a Medigap policy that provides the coverage you want, you do not have to switch to one of the new ones. And you may not want to change plans if your current policy pays for private rooms and private-duty nurses, and those amenities are important to you. Insurers no longer offer these coverages in the new policies.

If you are new to the Medigap market, first decide what optional coverages you want, if any. The following are some points to keep in mind when shopping for Medigap coverage.

Part B deductible. Buying deductible coverage to pay the first $100 of any physician or hospital outpatient charge is simply dollar trading. You may pay $100 in extra premiums for the coverage.

Part B excess charges. If your family doctor "takes assignment" (that is, accepts Medicare's allowable charge as payment in full), you may not need a policy that pays excess charges. However, that coverage could be useful if you someday need a team of specialists, some of whom do not take assignment.

At-home care after a hospital stay. If you currently own a long-term care policy that pays for home care, you will not need that coverage from a Medigap policy.

Prescription drugs. Drug coverage will be expensive, and you will still have a large out-of-pocket expense. If your current drug bill is less than the deductible, drug coverage may not pay off, at least right away. It might be useful if you need costlier drugs in the future.

Preventive medical care. This coverage may be unnecessary if you can cover the costs of flu vaccines and screening tests yourself.

Finally, buy no more than one policy. Find one that will give you all the protection you need.

HMOS FOR MEDICARE RECIPIENTS: SHOULD YOU JOIN?

Another option for Medicare-age people is to join a health maintenance organization. On the assumption that HMOs can deliver care more cheaply than conventional insurance plans, the U.S. government would like to see more Medicare recipients join HMOs in hopes of trimming its ever-growing Medicare bill.

For many older people, obtaining Medicare benefits from an HMO may be an appealing alternative to Medicare coverage and a traditional Medigap policy. It is likely to cost less, and an HMO may provide services that Medicare does not cover. But anyone considering joining a Medicare HMO had better be prepared to resist a hard, perhaps misleading, sales pitch.

At their best, some HMOs offer special programs

Does your Medicare cover as much as it should?

Not unless it offers 100% coverage. At no cost to you.* The federally approved CareFree Medicare Plan from CareFlorida makes sure you get no unexpected medical bills. No unwelcome surprises.

A simple call to 1-800-622-2734 starts the process. Under the CareFree Medicare Plan, your coverage includes:
- hearing aids
- prescription drugs
- eyeglasses
- routine check-ups in your choice of a private doctor's office or group practice
- dental services
- unlimited hospitalization
- emergency service
- catastrophic illnesses and much more.

With no deductibles, no co-payments, no monthly fees.

Give up the high cost of health care. Call today for a free information kit. With no obligation. We'll send you a magnifying glass just for calling. And, as you'll see, we can cover you in places you never dreamed of.

Easy Enrollment

CARE FLORIDA.
Don't worry. We cover it.
1-800-622-2734

In southern Florida, newspaper ads like this one from CareFlorida woo new customers with promises to cover what Medicare will not.

140

for Medicare members, screening them for illnesses after they join, directing them to preventive services, keeping track of the drugs they take, and making ombudspeople available to coordinate care and answer questions. At their worst, some HMOs make the elderly fight for benefits, especially the costly, skilled nursing or home care that plans must provide as part of the customary Medicare package of coverage. Some HMOs have dragged out the process of paying for these benefits so long that Medicare beneficiaries have died before ever receiving the nursing care they are legally entitled to.

HOW MEDICARE WORKS WITH HMOS

Before you even consider joining an HMO, you must understand the three ways Medicare pays HMOs to deliver care. These methods affect how members obtain medical services and what you pay for them.

1. *Risk contracts* take their name from the fact that the HMO assumes the financial risk of providing for a Medicare recipient's health care. Medicare pays the HMO a monthly sum to provide all the coverage for beneficiaries who join, much the same way an employer pays monthly premiums to provide all the care for its workers. (HMOs usually charge members a monthly premium calculated to cover the cost of Medicare deductibles and copayments.) The HMO is obligated to provide all the Part A (hospital) and Part B (medical) services.

In return, beneficiaries are "locked in" to the plan.

You cannot go outside, except for emergencies or urgently needed care away from the plan's service area. If you do, you must pay the bills yourself. Medicare will not reimburse you—a crucial point HMO salespeople often ignore.

Plans offering risk contracts must take all applicants regardless of their health, except those with end-stage kidney disease and those already in a Medicare hospice program. That is an advantage for older people who have serious medical problems.

2. *Cost contracts* are so named because they reimburse the HMO for the cost of providing care. Medicare pays a cost-contract HMO a fee to provide hospital and medical services. At the end of the year, if the plan spent more than Medicare has paid, Medicare reimburses the HMO. If an HMO has a cost contract, Medicare members are not locked in; you may obtain services outside the HMO network. Then, Medicare reimburses your expenses, and you will have to pay the usual copayments, deductibles, and extra physicians' charges you would normally pay had you not been in an HMO.

As with risk contracts, the HMO charges monthly premiums that cover Medicare deductibles and copayments. The HMO must take all older people who apply.

3. *Health-care prepayment plans* are plans under which Medicare pays the HMO to provide medical services only, not hospital services. The HMO does not have to cover all medical services but must provide for physicians' visits, X-rays, lab tests, and other diagnostic tests.

Beneficiaries can go outside the plan for any medical or hospital service. Again, if you do, you will receive regular Medicare benefits but must pay the deductibles, coinsurance, and extra charges that your doctors bill.

HMOs offering health-care prepayment plans can reject people in poor health. Unlike the other types of HMO plans, they are not required to have grievance procedures or quality-assurance programs.

The Ratings in Chapter 3 show which type of Medicare arrangement each rated HMO has made, and the monthly premiums for Medicare recipients. For all plans, beneficiaries must pay the 1992 monthly Medicare Part B premium of $31.80.

If you are willing to give up the family doctor, a risk plan offers the advantage of lower cost. Cost contracts and health-care prepayment plans give you flexibility to obtain medical care outside the plan. Doing that, however, could end up costing you a lot of money since you will have to pay Medicare copayments, deductibles, and excess physicians' charges each time you go elsewhere.

THE HARD SELL SURVIVES

HMOs actively solicit individual business only from those over 65. In some parts of the country, such as southern California and southern Florida, HMOs aggressively go after the Medicare market—nationally some 35 million men and women whose health care is paid for by the federal government.

Accustomed as *Consumer Reports* has become to insurance sales pitches, we were not surprised to find sales representatives who lied, omitted crucial information, and misled customers about their plans and even the Medicare program itself. We were, however, surprised at how pervasive the abuses were. In Miami Beach, our reporter sat in as a 65-year-old woman entertained representatives of AV-MED, CAC-Ramsay, Humana Medical Plan, PCA Health Plans, CareFlorida, and Health Options, an HMO operated by Blue Cross/Blue Shield of Florida. The presentations our reporter heard were as misleading as any she has witnessed.

The most grievous sales sin was failure to explain the "lock-in" feature that was part of each plan, an omission that could financially devastate an HMO member who went outside the network for care. Only the Humana salesperson emphasized that the woman would be required to get all her care from Humana doctors. However, he failed to tell her that she would not get Medicare benefits if she received care from a doctor outside the plan. None of the sales representatives could tell her anything meaningful about the physicians in their networks, but that hardly stopped them from picking a doctor for her. The Humana representative said he was not supposed to do that, but would do it anyway. He even offered to take the woman to look at the chosen doctor's office. The salesperson from Health Options steered her to a new doctor in the network, saying, "I like new doctors. They are not busy, and they like to please."

Most salespeople did a poor job of explaining Medicare. The business card for AV-MED's representative said he was a "Medicare consultant"; he barely mentioned how Medicare works. CareFlorida's "Medicare marketing representative" could not explain what Medicare meant by a "skilled nursing facility," saying only that it was licensed. Salespeople who hold themselves out as Medicare experts apparently are of no great concern to the Health Care Financing Administration (HCFA), which runs Medicare. The agency, for example, has no rules to prohibit HMO salespeople from using the term "Medicare consultant" on their business cards.

While they knew little about Medicare, the salespeople did have their hype down cold. Humana's salesperson described the plan as "the best in the country"—something the people we surveyed would strongly dispute. CAC-Ramsay's salesperson said his HMO "started the program and everyone followed us." And AV-MED's rep boasted, "AV-MED is not the Cadillac of HMOs. We're the Rolls Royce."

At the end, hyperbole and lies turned to old-fashioned high pressure. "I'm sorry you're not making up your mind. You'll regret it. Don't get involved with anyone else," warned the salesperson from Health Options. "You make me look bad with the company," said PCA's representative when the woman did not sign up on the spot. The clincher came from the representatives of CAC-Ramsay. Its front office later calls new members to make sure that they understand the plan. "When the girls call to verify, don't ask any questions," the salesperson warned. "That means you don't understand the program, and we'll have to come back and explain it."

WHO'S WATCHING THE HMOS?

Joining an HMO can be tricky—and not just because the salespeople are of so little help. The government's payment scheme is confusing and its oversight of the HMO industry lackadaisical. *Consumer Reports* looked at enrollment and disenrollment data collected by the Health Care Financing Administration (HCFA) and found large numbers of beneficiaries leaving certain plans. Take Humana Medical Plan of South Florida, an HMO that has come under severe criticism for its dealings with older people. In 1990, Humana enrolled nearly 69,000 new members, but more than 31,000 dropped out. In 1991, the plan enrolled 54,000 and 33,000 left.

HCFA cautions against putting too much emphasis on such statistics, since high disenrollments do not necessarily mean an HMO's members are unhappy. Our respondents seemed to say otherwise. Humana was one of the lowest-ranked HMOs. Furthermore, at the time of the enrollments, Humana was not in compliance with certain federal requirements; for that reason, the U.S. General Accounting Office said HCFA should not have let new members sign up there. (HCFA can suspend an HMO's authority to enroll new beneficiaries.)

We also looked at government data on the number of complaints that Medicare recipients made to HCFA about the HMOs we rated (see Ratings in Chapter 3). Two plans stood out for the volume of complaints they generated. During 1990 and 1991,

Medicare recipients filed more than 7,000 complaints about Humana Medical Plan, a large number even for a large HMO. They also filed more than 4,000 complaints about Foundation Health Plan, an HMO about average in *Consumer Reports'* survey. PacifiCare, which ranked below average in our survey, had the next highest number of complaints—947.

Again, the HCFA maintains that the complaint statistics, like the disenrollment statistics, are not meaningful. If so, the agency has done little to make its data more useful. Nor does the agency routinely check for the quality of care delivered by all the HMOs it contracts with or act against the dishonest and misleading sales presentations like those our reporter observed. So it's not surprising that the General Accounting Office has found "persistent problems with some HMOs' compliance with Medicare requirements."

5
LONG-TERM CARE INSURANCE

*"Some consumer abuses are so
severe as to raise questions
about the very viability of this
product."*

L ong-term care insurance promises to pay the
bills if you need to enter a nursing home or
be cared for at your own home. But our 1991
survey of long-term care policies raises serious questions about their ability to make good on that promise.

Forty-three percent of all Americans who turn 65
this year will eventually enter a nursing home. Twenty-five percent of that group will stay at least one

year, at a cost of $30,000 to $40,000. By the year 2010, the cost of a year's stay in a nursing home could easily top $83,000. Some people will pay their entire bill with money they have saved. Others will begin paying with their own savings, then turn to Medicaid when their money runs out. Still others will rely on Medicaid from the beginning. A few will use the proceeds from an insurance policy.

Insurance companies are pushing consumers to buy long-term care policies. And government officials are eager to cut Medicaid spending. The evidence suggests they are succeeding. More than 1.5 million policies had been sold as of 1991 (up from 815,000 in 1987). Some 140 companies now offer coverage, either as a separate policy or as part of a life insurance contract (up from 75 companies in 1987). But behind the sales statistics are signs of serious trouble. Some people are spending thousands of dollars a year for coverage. But many insurers are betting, perhaps hoping, that their customers will drop the policies before collecting a penny in benefits. Furthermore, poorly trained and sometimes unscrupulous agents are seriously misleading buyers about the terms, benefits, and limitations of their coverage.

The policies themselves, though somewhat improved since *Consumer Reports* first examined them in 1988, still have significant shortcomings. The following are among the traps awaiting consumers:

- Confusing policy language
- Tricky provisions in the way policies are written
- The potential for unaffordably large rate increases
- Uncertainty about whether claims will be paid.

150

Since 1988, insurers have created a dizzying array of new policies, riders, and features. Almost every policy is different from every other policy. Even a number of insurance regulators who encouraged the development of the market are having second thoughts. "Some consumer abuses are so severe as to raise questions about the very viability of this product," Earl Pomeroy, past president of the National Association of Insurance Commissioners, told *Consumer Reports*.

QUALIFYING FOR MEDICAID

Through Medicaid, the federal–state program that finances medical care for the poor, the government has provided something of a long-term care safety net. Medicaid currently covers about half of all nursing-home stays. To qualify for Medicaid, a patient's assets cannot exceed a maximum amount specified by the state. Depending on the state, between 25 and 52 percent of all people admitted to a nursing home turn to Medicaid right away. Another 4 to 18 percent become eligible later during their nursing-home confinement, after their bills have reduced them to the ranks of the poor.

The process by which medical and nursing-home care reduces a person's assets is called a "spend-down." Once eligible for Medicaid, a nursing-home patient with no spouse or dependents must turn over to the nursing facility all of his or her income, including Social Security checks, except for a small personal-needs allowance of $30 to $50 a month. Here's how a spend-down works: Suppose an elderly widow

151

living in New York City requires a long nursing-home stay. She has $25,000 in bank certificates of deposit. Her annual income from Social Security, pension, and interest comes to $15,000, or $1,250 a month.

Nursing homes in her area cost about $5,000 a month, so her monthly income is insufficient to cover the expense. She will eventually need help from Medicaid. However, when she enters the nursing home, her $25,000 in assets will exceed New York's asset limit for a single person—namely, $3,000. When she first enters the nursing home, she must spend $1,200 of her monthly income on her care. (Again, she can keep $50 for personal needs.) To cover the rest of her nursing-home expenses, she has to draw down her savings. When she has spent $20,500 of her $25,000, she can turn to Medicaid for help. She can keep the remaining $4,500 (the $3,000 asset allowance plus another $1,500 for burial expenses). Her income and savings will buy about five months of care before Medicaid steps in.

"Two ways to protect your assets from being consumed by a Medicare spend-down: estate-planning devices and long-term care insurance."

After she depletes her assets, she will continue to apply her monthly income to nursing-home costs, but Medicaid will pay the balance of the monthly charge.

For married couples, a spend-down once meant poverty for a nursing-home resident's spouse who remained at home. Congress has since made it somewhat easier for spouses to maintain a decent, if modest, standard of living.

Each state determines how much of a couple's assets the spouse at home can keep. The federal government, however, sets limits. These range from a minimum of $13,740 in 1992 to a maximum of $68,700. When a couple's assets are under $13,740, the spouse at home can keep the entire amount. (The applicant's home, household goods, and personal effects are not counted.) The spouse at home can continue to live in the family house. However, the state can recoup what its Medicaid program has spent after both spouses die. States also dictate how much income the spouse not in the the nursing home can have. No state can set a limit lower than $985 a month or one higher than $1,718 in 1992. Both asset and income limits are adjusted each year for inflation.

PROTECTING YOUR ASSETS

There are two ways to protect your assets from being consumed by a Medicare spend-down. One is to use estate-planning devices, such as making outright gifts of money to family members or setting up a specific kind of trust. You will need the help of a lawyer if you decide to do this. You can also be sure that Medicaid will carefully review your arrangements to see if you followed the rules. If you want to transfer assets, you must do so at least 30 months before applying for Medicaid. If you transfer your assets for less than their fair market value, and if the transfer occurs less than 30 months before you go to a nursing home, you will be temporarily ineligible for Medicaid, for a period of up to 30 months.

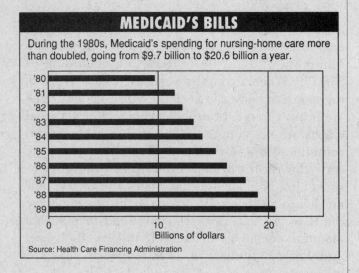

MEDICAID'S BILLS

During the 1980s, Medicaid's spending for nursing-home care more than doubled, going from $9.7 billion to $20.6 billion a year.

'80
'81
'82
'83
'84
'85
'86
'87
'88
'89

0   10   20

Billions of dollars

Source: Health Care Financing Administration

The time limit does not apply if you receive care in your home or in a Medicaid-approved facility, such as an adult day-care center that provides medical treatment. Under those circumstances, you can transfer your assets one day and Medicaid will begin paying for your care the next.

The other asset-protection method is to purchase long-term care insurance.

LONG-TERM CARE POLICIES

Insurance companies sell three kinds of long-term care policies: Those that cover only nursing-home stays; those that cover only care at home; and those that cover both. Some life-insurance policies have riders that pay for long-term care; those are not discussed here.

154

Nursing-home coverage. Typically, this means all levels of nursing care—skilled, intermediate, and custodial. Skilled care is intensive, round-the-clock medical care by trained, licensed personnel. Intermediate care is similar but less intensive. Custodial (or personal) care helps patients with everyday activities such as eating, bathing, dressing, and moving about.

Unlike older policies, the current crop cover all three levels of nursing care, and most make no distinction among them, simply saying that they will pay for any nursing care a person needs. But beware: The policyholder still may not collect benefits. A company can deny a claim if care is not provided in what it defines as an eligible facility.

Home-care coverage. When you think of "home care," you may envision someone coming to a person's house to prepare meals, clean, help with dressing, and run a few errands. It's not that simple; most insurance companies do not interpret "home care" that way. A few pay home-care benefits only for skilled nursing care performed by registered nurses, licensed practical nurses, and occupational, speech, or physical therapists. Others cover the services of home health aides employed by licensed agencies. Such aides have less training and primarily help patients with personal or custodial care. A policy that covers home health aides is obviously more desirable than one that pays only for skilled personnel. Better still are policies that pay for homemaker services— cooking, cleaning, and running errands. Only a few

155

companies, however, offer this benefit, and some of those limit how much they will pay. Several others are willing to pay home health aides to do a little house-keeping, so long as they also provide personal care.

Policies do not pay benefits to family members who perform home-care services. If you buy a long-term care policy, don't count on the insurance company someday paying your granddaughter to help out.

A few policies offer what are called recuperative, home again, or post-confinement benefits, usually as a substitute for real home-care coverage. These are of limited value since they typically pay only for a short period following a nursing-home or hospital stay.

Other provisions. Certain long-term care policies offer distinctive features.

Waiver of premium, for instance, allows the policy-holder to stop paying premiums during a nursing-home stay, once the company has begun paying benefits. A few companies waive the premium as soon as a policyholder receives the first payment. But waits of between 60 and 90 days are more typical. Most do not waive premiums if the policyholder receives nursing care at home.

Nonforfeiture benefits return to policyholders some of their equity if they drop their coverage. Without that benefit, if you drop the policy after 10 or 20 years, your loss could be sizable. To minimize such losses, policyholders may also be able to buy a policy with a "reduced paid-up" arrangement, in which part of the benefits are payable after the policy is dropped. Other carriers may offer a "return of premium" non-

forfeiture benefit, under which they return all or a portion of the premiums after a certain number of years, if the policyholder decides to drop the policy. Nonforfeiture benefits are not common in individual policies. They are more likely to be found as an option in group plans offered through employers.

Death benefits refund to the policyholder's estate any premiums paid (minus any benefits the company paid on the policyholder's behalf). This benefit is usually payable only if the policyholder dies before a certain age, typically 65 or 70.

BEING IN THE RIGHT PLACE

With long-term care policies, the type of facility where services are performed can mean the difference between receiving payment on a claim or having the claim denied.

Nursing-home coverage. The most liberal coverage, Consumers Union believes, would be provided by policies that allowed policyholders to obtain services wherever they wished when they were disabled. Once policyholders qualified for benefits, the company would simply give them the money to spend.

All other policies are "service based"; that means policyholders must obtain services from providers that meet qualifications set by the insurance company. Some of these policies are more liberal than others. The best of them pay for care in any licensed facility. But the majority of policies are more restrictive, particularly in the area of custodial care, the kind most people are likely to need.

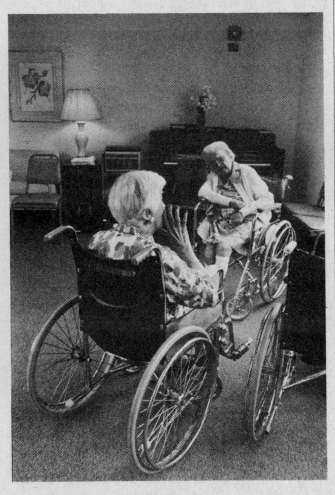

A year's stay in a nursing home averages about $30,000. By the year 2010, it could easily top $83,000.

Policies that limit custodial services do so in several ways. Many will not cover custodial care unless it's provided in a skilled- or intermediate-nursing facility.

Other policies say they cover custodial care, but go on to exclude, by name, some types of facilities that are licensed to provide it. For example, most policies will not pay for custodial services in homes for the aged, although such homes are licensed to provide custodial care in several states.

Still other carriers use the fine print in their contracts to restrict coverage. A policy may, for instance, only pay for care in a custodial facility that has at least 25 residents. But in Arizona and Oregon, for example, custodial facilities legally may care for fewer people than that. Policyholders in those states may be out of luck if they happen to be in the wrong custodial facility. Or a policy may require custodial facilities to provide continuous nursing services under the supervision of a physician or a graduate registered nurse. But in Pennsylvania, homes that provide custodial care do not need supervisory nurses on duty.

Home-care coverage. As its name implies, most home care is given in a policyholder's residence. But the more generous policies also allow policyholders to receive benefits in adult day-care centers. Such policies may, however, define the term "adult day-care center" more restrictively than certain states do, effectively preventing policyholders in some state-approved facilities from collecting benefits.

GETTING PAST THE GATES

All policies have "gatekeepers"—restrictions that determine who is eligible to receive benefits. These gatekeepers are the most important feature of a policy, but the one buyers hear least about. And no wonder: Even agents do not understand them, because few companies teach agents how they work. Outlines of coverage (a document summarizing the policy provisions) seldom discuss them, and sales brochures are usually silent as well.

Under the least restrictive, and rarest, policies, a policyholder qualifies for benefits if his or her doctor orders the care. More common are restrictive policies that require care to be medically necessary for sickness or injury. Yet many nursing-home patients, especially those needing only custodial care, are not sick or injured; they may not qualify for benefits under a policy with this gatekeeper. Furthermore, the standard is subjective. A company may liberally interpret it today, but several years from now, after experiencing costly claims, the carrier could argue that a stay is not "medically necessary."

A third type of gatekeeper requires policyholders to be unable to perform a certain number of "activities of daily living" (commonly referred to as ADLs) before the company will pay benefits. The activities usually include bathing, dressing, eating, using the toilet, walking, maintaining continence, taking medicine, and transferring from bed to chair. Sometimes a company with an "activities" standard also allows policyholders who fail certain mental (or cognitive) tests to qualify for benefits.

A policyholder may have an easier time qualifying under a policy with an "activities" standard than under a policy requiring sickness or injury. Nevertheless, such a standard can be restrictive. Most policies define "activities of daily living" vaguely, leaving the final decision in each individual case to a company claims analyst. Only a few policies thoroughly explain what they mean by failure to perform an activity, a practice we believe other carriers should adopt.

Policies differ about which activities, and how many, policyholders must be unable to perform before they are eligible for benefits. A few policies require that policyholders be unable to perform activities of daily living specifically because of sickness or injury. That is the most restrictive gatekeeper.

Even though state regulators require all policies to cover Alzheimer's disease, policyholders with the disease may be denied benefits if they are physically able to perform the activities of daily living. If a company uses an activities standard to judge whether the policyholder is entitled to benefits, and if it does not specifically allow people whose only problem is severe memory loss to qualify, patients with Alzheimer's disease may not be covered. Only a minority of policies in our study had a separate gatekeeper involving cognitive tests.

Long-term care policies may still include the requirement of a hospital stay of at least three days before the company will pay nursing-home benefits. That requirement is illegal in 43 states, and we recommend avoiding policies that contain it.

BENEFITS BASICS

Insurance companies offer policyholders a choice of daily benefits for nursing-home care that typically range from $40 to $120. If home-care coverage is

Inflation Protection

A 65-year-old who buys a long-term care policy today may not need it for 20 years. A nursing home that currently costs $86 a day could cost $228 a day 20 years from now, assuming a relatively modest inflation rate of 5 percent a year. Such statistics underscore the importance of securing good inflation protection in a long-term care policy. Unfortunately, the companies that told *Consumer Reports* what percentage of their policies are sold with inflation protection reported that only half their policyholders adopted it. We think buyers who forgo good inflation protection are ill-advised.

Not all inflation protection provisions are created equally. Insurers use two methods to increase coverage to account for inflation. One method lets policyholders buy additional coverage every few years at the then-current price, based on their age at that time. Usually they do not have to prove that they are still insurable. The price of that additional coverage, however, can go up so rapidly it will become virtually unaffordable. And policyholders who do not buy the additional benefits when offered may lose their right to buy more in the future.

The second method is somewhat more realistic. It automatically increases the daily benefit by some percentage each year, usually 5 percent, uncompounded. A typical $80 benefit that increases 5 percent a year will be worth $160 in 20 years. An $80 benefit compounded at 5 percent would be worth $212 in 20 years.

Unfortunately, most companies do not offer compounded inflation protection. Only a few companies offer inflation protection that will continue as long as the policy stays in force. Most others discontinue inflation increases after 10 or 20 years, regardless of the method they use. A few companies discontinue them when a policyholder reaches age 80 or 85, just the age when someone is most likely to go to a nursing home. People who purchase a long-term care policy at age 55 or 60 (when companies most want them to buy) may discover that their ability to increase coverage has ended long before they will need nursing care—in effect freezing their benefits at an inadequate level.

Good inflation protection is expensive. It can add between 25 and 40 percent to the premium, and sometimes more. Some companies using the automatic-increase approach charge a level premium for the inflation rider even though the benefit goes up each year. Others increase the premium at the same rate as the benefit; that is, 5 percent a year. If the latter is the case, beware. Those riders may cost less to begin with, but they may eventually become more expensive than you can afford, perhaps forcing you to drop your coverage just when you are most likely to need it.

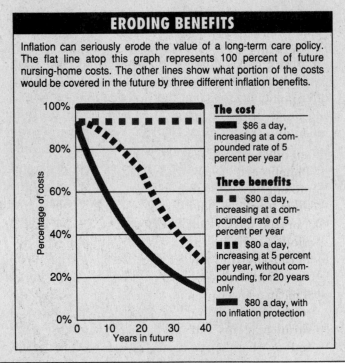

ERODING BENEFITS

Inflation can seriously erode the value of a long-term care policy. The flat line atop this graph represents 100 percent of future nursing-home costs. The other lines show what portion of the costs would be covered in the future by three different inflation benefits.

The cost

■■ $86 a day, increasing at a compounded rate of 5 percent per year

Three benefits

■ ■ $80 a day, increasing at a compounded rate of 5 percent per year

■■■ $80 a day, increasing at 5 percent per year, without compounding, for 20 years only

■ $80 a day, with no inflation protection

sold as part of the policy, the dollar benefit is often half that for nursing-home care.

Home-care-only policies pay up to a fixed daily amount, or up to a fixed number of dollars per hour, of service ($50 a day or $15 an hour, for example). A few policies do not limit the daily amounts, but instead set a lifetime dollar maximum for policyholders to use as needed; $50,000 is typical. Policies generally pay nursing-home benefits for a minimum of one year. Insurers also offer two-, three-, four-, five-, and six-year plans. Others will pay for as long as 10 years or for the rest of a policyholder's life. While most nursing-home stays are short—the average is only 19 months—longer coverage can protect policyholders and their families against the financial ravages of a catastrophic illness that might go on for several years. When home care is combined with nursing-home coverage, the home-care benefit period is sometimes shorter than that for a nursing-home stay. With home-care-only plans, benefit periods are often one to two years.

Benefits can start as soon as the policyholder enters a nursing home, or they can begin after a "waiting," "elimination," or "deductible" period of 20, 30, 60, 90, or 100 days. Some policies have shorter waiting periods for home-care benefits. For policyholders who can afford to pay for several days or months of care from their own savings, a longer waiting period can mean a lower premium. We found, however, that often consumers are given little choice. Instead, insurance agents will make the selection for them, based on what that particular company wants to sell.

ARE YOU INSURABLE?

Not everyone who applies for a policy gets one. Your chances depend on your health and on how carefully a company checks it. Some insurers put little effort into screening applicants and take on almost all comers. Others reject as many as 40 percent of those who apply.

All companies' applications ask whether the applicant has had certain conditions, such as cancer, heart disease, Alzheimer's disease, or osteoporosis. They may also ask if the applicant has seen a doctor in the last year and if he or she uses a wheelchair. At companies that do little checking, a "yes" answer to any of the health questions will automatically disqualify an applicant. The agent may not even submit the application to the home office. But if applicants answer "no" to every question, their coverage may begin within days. However, when those policyholders submit a claim, the company may then look at their medical histories to make sure they told the truth on their applications. If they lied (even with an agent's tacit consent), the insurer can deny their claims, cancel their policies, and return the premiums they have paid. This onerous practice is called "post-claims underwriting."

Companies that conduct more careful reviews will investigate your health history before issuing a policy. The company may ask for a doctor's statement or for all your medical records over a specified period of time.

Generally, companies do not want to insure people who have had strokes, diabetes, multiple sclerosis, recent cancer surgery, asthma, macular degeneration (an eye disease), severe high blood pressure, or

166

Will Your Claim Be Paid?

Insurance carriers rarely pay all the claims their policyholders submit. *Consumer Reports* tried to find out what portion of claims they do pay, but most companies would not say.

Data that companies did share indicate that a large number of claims are turned down, often because policyholders do not understand the limitations lacing their contracts. One company reported that in 1989 it denied 80 percent of the claims made under its home-care-only policy. Another told us it turned down about a third of the claims submitted. A third company refused 22 percent of its claims.

Alzheimer's disease. But some companies are more selective than others. For example, one company may not cover someone who has had hip-replacement surgery within the last 18 months; another will.

Some insurers will accept people with health problems but will charge them more or offer slimmer benefits. How much extra applicants with health problems will have to pay depends on both the severity of their ailments and on the insurer. A severe illness might mean a doubling of the standard rate, while a milder one would result in only a 15-percent increase.

Insurers also differ in how they handle "pre-existing conditions," health problems policyholders had when they purchased their policy. Some insurers make policyholders wait six months before they will cover pre-existing conditions. Others impose no waiting period. Insurers that carefully check an applicant's health before issuing a policy are more likely not to impose a waiting period.

Some companies also have "preferred" rates for applicants who are in better health or meet certain other conditions. But the rates labeled "preferred," "standard," and "substandard" are not comparable across companies. A preferred rate at one company may be the standard rate at another.

THE COSTS: TODAY AND TOMORROW

Long-term care insurance is not cheap. A 65-year-old can expect to pay around $1,000 a year to most companies for a policy with both nursing-home and home-care coverage; a 75-year-old will pay upward of $2,000. Prices vary considerably among carriers. An $80 benefit payable for four years with a 30-day waiting period could cost a 65-year-old as much as $3,020 or as little as $766. Not surprisingly, the larger the benefit, the longer it lasts; and the sooner it begins, the higher the price. Inflation protection can add $1,000 or more to the premium, and home-care coverage another $150 to $600.

Home-care-only policies are somewhat cheaper. A 65-year-old could pay as much as $675 or as little as $254 for a policy from the companies in our 1991 survey.

"The next five years will produce rate increases, as the rule rather than the exception, for most companies currently marketing long-term care insurance."

All long-term care policies are guaranteed renewable. But though a carrier must renew your coverage every year, it does not have to guarantee the rates you will pay. Most policies have "level" premiums—that is, they don't rise with the policyholder's age. However, premiums can rise across the board for all policyholders if an insurer experiences more claims expense than it anticipated. The policy with the lowest price today may well turn out to be the worst buy later on. "The next five years will produce rate increases, as the rule rather than the exception, for most companies currently marketing long-term care insurance," Barry Grove, a vice president and actuary with Standard Life and Accident, told *Consumer Reports* in 1991. Companies may initially offer lower premiums and higher benefit levels to stimulate sales, but such a recipe for today's sales success may be tomorrow's prescription for disaster. Companies can justify lower premiums by underestimating the dollar value of claims they will eventually have to pay or by overestimating the number of policyholders who will drop their coverage before they ever file a claim. Some insurers are doing both. Either way, if more claims materialize than the company has counted on, it will have to raise policyholders' premiums or risk insolvency.

The case of United Equitable shows what can happen when a company miscalculates. In the early 1980s, United Equitable was one of the largest sellers of long-term care insurance, with some 60,000 policyholders. When those policyholders began to make claims in big numbers, it became clear that the company had underpriced its policies. Policyholders were staying in nursing homes longer and running up far higher bills than the company had anticipated when it priced the policies. In 1986, Standard Life and Accident took over United Equitable's policies and raised premiums by 103 to 213 percent. Most policyholders dropped their coverage as a result. Of the original 60,000 policyholders, only about 12,000 were left by 1991.

SALES PITCHES: ETHICAL POLICY LAPSES

Midway through a 1990 sales pitch, a California insurance agent representing Pioneer Life pulled a copy of the June 1989 *Consumer Reports* from his briefcase and displayed our article on Medicare-supplement insurance. He pointed to his company's number-two ranking. "*Consumer Reports* rated this policy number two out of the top 50 companies writing nursing-home insurance," he said proudly. But Medicare-supplement insurance and nursing-home insurance are two completely different products, as any good insurance agent would know. That agent either did not know, or did not want the truth to interfere with his sales pitch. Nor did he know that he was talking to the very *Consumer Reports* staffer who had written the article. "Number two for *nursing-home* insurance?" she asked him, just to make sure he had not made an innocent mistake.

"Yes," the agent assured her. Then he proceeded to show how good his company was by knocking the top-rated carrier, claiming its policy was sold only through a teachers' association—another of the many falsehoods that laced his sales presentation. Bad as he was, that agent was far from unique in his willingness to mislead and confuse. Our reporter, who posed as a relative of an elderly shopper for long-term care insurance, listened to 14 other sales presentations in California, Florida, and New York by agents representing some of the largest sellers of that coverage—American Integrity, AMEX Life, CNA, Medico, Penn Treaty, Pioneer Life, John Hancock, and Transport Life. She heard lies, she witnessed ignorance or deceit, and she saw ethical standards violated and state law ignored.

Every sales agent misrepresented some aspect of

the policy, the financial condition of the insurer, or the quality of a competitor's product. Not one sales agent properly explained the benefits, restrictions, and policy limitations. Almost all, for example, failed to discuss the policies' gatekeepers, those vital provisions that govern whether a policyholder will actually collect benefits.

Some agents' pitches were far too brief to be of real value. Those agents highlighted a few obvious points from a sales brochure and skipped the more arcane but important ones. For instance, a Pioneer Life salesman in Florida noted that his policy paid for ambulance rides (an insignificant benefit), but did not tell the prospective buyer that her premiums would increase as she got older, an onerous feature that, in our opinion, makes a policy unacceptable. Other pitches were far too long. Agents settled into their chairs as if prepared to stay forever and told story after scary story about people who did not buy.

Not only did agents fail to explain their policies properly, they left behind no written information that would. In violation of their states' insurance laws, 11 of the 15 agents did not provide outlines of coverage or disclosure statements for all the policies they were selling. And not one left the shoppers' guide written by the National Association of Insurance Commissioners. The guide must be delivered at the time an insurance agent comes calling. None produced sample policies when asked for them. "Sample policies don't mean a thing," said a representative of Transport Life. However, all left sketchy brochures which, one agent insisted, "tell more than the policy."

Long-term care policies are the most complicated of all individual insurance products. But if ever there was a product that consumers were asked to buy blindly, this is it.

AFFORDABILITY?

Long-term care insurance is not for everyone. Only those who can afford to pay the premiums for many years and who have substantial assets to protect should even consider a policy.

Any responsible sales agent should first assess whether a client needs the coverage and can afford it. Only one agent in our test asked about his customer's finances, but he then paid no attention to what she told him. The customer, a retired school teacher who had only $10,000 in assets and who would have qualified for MediCal (California's version of Medicaid) within a few months of entering a nursing home, was not a candidate for long-term care insurance. Nevertheless, the agent did not hesitate to use the hard sell. "They trained me in sales to get five no's before leaving," he told her. He got them.

An AMEX Life agent pushed his policy on a 72-year-old woman for more than two hours without asking a single question about her finances. In doing so, he ignored his own company's code of ethics, which requires him to sell only to "customers whose financial position allows them to consider purchasing long-term care insurance."

Agents selling long-term care insurance are, however, quick to adapt their pitch to how much they think their sales prospect can afford to pay. Transport Life has instructed its agents: "Through the use of different daily benefits and benefit periods, there is a plan to match almost any budget. The key is to match their budget!" Agents for Transport and other companies consistently pursued that sales strategy. One Transport agent who initially pitched an $80 daily benefit effortlessly shifted to a $60 plan when one woman balked at the price. "It's a whole bunch better to have $1,800 a month [$60 x 30 days] than to be not covered. Anything is better than nothing," the agent said, desperate to make a sale. However, nursing-home costs in the woman's area were currently running about $100 a day. By the time she needed nursing care at, say, age 85—13 years later—the daily charges would be about $189 (assuming a 5 percent annual increase in nursing-home costs). The $60 benefit would then provide $1,800 a month, and leave $3,870 a month unpaid.

" 'Anything is better than nothing,' the agent said, desperate to make a sale."

An American Integrity agent recommended "at least an $80 benefit," but urged his prospect to take $90. When the woman said she could not pay the $1,304 premium, he responded, "If I were to use one of the other carriers, we'd be looking at $2,000." When that didn't change her mind, he finally said: "Do something, even if you take only $70."

To keep premiums low and the products "affordable," most agents our reporter listened to discouraged buyers from purchasing inflation riders that automatically increase benefits. A John Hancock agent simply crossed off the inflation rider from the sales brochure and said it was unavailable in New York. The home office in Boston said otherwise. "It's an integral part of the policy and was approved in New York," Gail Schaeffer, a Hancock vice president, told *Consumer Reports*.

The few agents who mentioned the riders did a poor job of explaining them. Our reporter asked an agent for Gerber Life and American Integrity if his company's inflation benefits compounded every year. "It just increases up to 10 years," he replied, either ducking the question or not understanding the mysteries of compounding. A CNA agent assured our reporter that his company's rider *was* compounded. CNA's sales brochure said it was not.

Nowhere was the fog thicker than in the area of home-care coverage. Home-care benefits vary greatly from policy to policy, making it hard for buyers to grope their way through the maze of provisions. Agents made the task even harder. Frequently they misrepresented the coverage, leading prospective buyers to believe they would be covered for more services than was true. A Florida agent pushing Medico's home-care policy tried to sell a $100 daily benefit instead of a $70 plan. "If you go above $70, you can get people to come in and clean," he advised. "I have a lot of clients who like someone to change their sheets and comb their hair. You're not going to get that for $70 a day. A $70 benefit buys only the medical things; $100 allows the agency to give you some things for health and comfort." In fact, policyholders may not get their sheets changed, vacuuming done, or hair combed, even for $100. According to a sales brochure the agent left, the policy covers only "nursing-care services and . . . medical and health-related services . . . prescribed by a physician."

A Transport Life agent in Florida said his policy would pay for someone "to come in, clean house, and fix meals. It pays for housekeeping, and it pays forever." An official at Transport's home office in Dallas told a different story: "If a home health aide does a little vacuuming, we don't quibble. If they bring in a homemaker, a chauffeur, or a go-fer, it's not covered."

Agents were not so eager to tell prospective buyers that their premiums might increase. Premiums can go up if insurers raise them for everyone who has bought the same policy. We believe large rate increases may be in store for many policyholders.

A Transport Life agent told his prospect, "The rates you'll pay today are the rates you'll pay forever. This plan locks in the rate." To reassure her, he pointed to the company's sales brochure and said, "It tells you so there." When our reporter later reviewed the brochure, she found that, contrary to the agent's assertion, rates could go up, although the company played down the possibility by using the word "change" rather than "increase."

AND THE PITCH GOES ON

Another subject agents preferred to avoid was the state of their prospect's health. Though many insurance carriers tell agents to weed out people in bad

health before submitting applications to the home office, we found that agents often ignore company rules. One California agent selling for Pioneer Life told his prospect that she was eligible for the company's "preferred" rate without even asking her three questions required by his company. Instead he simply said, "You have no Alzheimer's or heart problems, do you?" and moved on with his pitch. Another agent who represented several carriers asked no questions about his prospect's health. "She's 100 percent insurable. I can tell by looking at her," he said. The woman suffered from macular degeneration, an eye disease that, in fact, would make her uninsurable at many companies as soon as they had checked her medical history.

Agents gave their most absurd answers when asked about their companies' financial stability and what would happen to a policyholder if the insurer went under. A Medico agent in California said, "Not one insurance company can really fold. Every company has to have assets and liabilities. The state of California sees to that." He did not say what happens if the liabilities someday exceed the assets.

A Medico agent in Florida offered this reassurance: "Insurance companies go out of business. It happens every day. All that went out were D-rated companies." However, A.M. Best, the best-known organization that rates the financial condition of insurance companies, does not give D ratings. And even A-rated companies do go out of business sometimes.

An AMEX Life agent said his company was in good financial shape because it used to be owned by The Travelers, one of the country's largest insurers. Not

so, the president of AMEX later told us; the company was never part of The Travelers.

Then there was the Pioneer agent who said of his company, "I don't think they are going to go out of business. The biggest problem we have is that they are in Rockford, Illinois, and the mail doesn't get there that fast"!

As sales pitches drew to a close and prospects said they wanted to do some further shopping, some agents resorted to knocking the competition. An American Integrity salesperson warned his prospect to stay away from a competing product because "their coverage is very expensive." That company's premiums were reasonably high, but, again, policies with the lowest prices may not be worth buying.

One CNA agent did not discourse about his competitors but gave his prospect the name of an official at the Florida Insurance Department and suggested she call him for a reference. Later we asked the Florida Insurance Department about that. It told us that it does not "give personal opinions about agents."

Though every state regulates insurance companies, do not rely on the government to protect you against misleading sales pitches.

We found numerous instances where sales brochures and even outlines of coverage could mislead buyers about how the policies actually worked. In their defense it must be added that state regulators are overwhelmed by the sheer number of policies, their many themes and variations, and by the lack of staff to sort them all out.

REGULATORY ROULETTE

The National Association of Insurance Commissioners (NAIC), the group that writes model laws for all states to adopt, has tried to cure obvious defects in long-term care policies. But as soon as it fixes one, another pops up. Among the current problems are the following:

- The NAIC passed a model law that has virtually eliminated requirements for a three-day hospital stay before the policy pays benefits. Yet it still allows companies to use other restrictions that could turn out to be just as harsh.
- The NAIC model regulations require companies to cover Alzheimer's disease, but they permit them to use eligibility standards that may actually prevent some Alzheimer's patients from receiving benefits.
- The model requires policies to cover more than just skilled nursing care, but companies may still deny coverage if that care is not given in the right type of facility.
- The NAIC-designed financial statement that insurance companies must file annually requires them to report data about the premiums they collect and claims they pay for long-term care policies. However, some states may not be penalizing companies that do not comply.

When our reporter visited the Florida Insurance Department, she found that several companies had failed to file the required NAIC information due 10 months earlier. Until she inquired, regulators had not noticed the forms were missing.

Even when the NAIC has proposed model laws to police the industry, states have been slow to adopt them. Only 25 states prohibit the onerous practice of *post-claims underwriting,* by which a company decides whether you were eligible to buy insurance at the time you make a claim rather than at the time it sells you a policy.

Only 29 states have standards for home-care benefits. And only 31 states protect buyers of group policies by giving them the right to continue their coverage on an individual basis when they leave the group.

"In post-claims underwriting, a company decides whether you were eligible to buy insurance at the time you make a claim rather than at the time it sells you a policy."

To promote the growth of long-term care insurance, the NAIC has allowed carriers the freedom to innovate and create new products. But that freedom has produced policies so complex that it is virtually impossible for consumers to decipher and compare them.

Also to encourage growth, the NAIC has tried to keep premiums "affordable." Regulators have been reluctant to mandate expensive, but worthwhile, coverages, such as inflation protection and nonforfeiture benefits. Without inflation protection, the value of the benefit will shrink dangerously by the time a policyholder needs care. Without nonforfeiture benefits, policyholders will lose their entire equity in the policy if they cannot afford to keep paying premiums.

THE INSOLVENCY QUESTION

As if misleading sales claims were not enough to worry about, buyers of long-term care insurance have no guarantee that the company they select will be around when they need it. In June 1990, for instance, the Oregon Department of Insurance shut down Farwest American Assurance, a major life and health insurer in the Northwest, and began to distribute its assets to pay claims and creditors. Two years earlier, that company had earned a more-than-respectable A rating from A.M. Best, the authority on insurance-company finances.

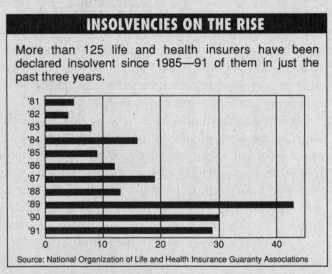

INSOLVENCIES ON THE RISE

More than 125 life and health insurers have been declared insolvent since 1985—91 of them in just the past three years.

Source: National Organization of Life and Health Insurance Guaranty Associations

Farwest American's long-term care policy had also earned a more-than-respectable quality rating from *Consumer Reports*, ranking in the top quarter of the policies we rated in 1988. Consumers had little reason to doubt the financial stability of Farwest American. A.M. Best had awarded the company an A rating since 1976, and in its 1988 report, Best noted that the premiums the company collected had increased more than 530 percent in the most recent five-year period. Insurance regulators suspected no trouble; quarterly financial reports the company had been filing with them appeared to be in order.

That picture of financial tranquility changed very quickly. In early 1989, First Farwest Life, the parent company of Farwest American Assurance, advised Oregon insurance regulators that it was insolvent. The liabilities of First Farwest Life and *its* own parent, the National Hospital Association, exceeded assets by some $14 million. Regulators then liquidated the assets of both parent companies to pay claims. At the same time, regulators tried to salvage Farwest American, but they were unsuccessful.

Farwest American and First Farwest Life had both been selling long-term care policies. But like many other sellers of long-term care insurance, their main line of business was group major–medical coverage. And like many sellers of major–medical coverage, they had underpriced their policies. The rapid escalation of health-care costs in the late 1980s doomed both carriers. The companies had collected insufficient premiums to pay the claims that began to pile up.

One-quarter of the companies whose policies we rated in 1988 were no longer selling long-term care insurance the next time we looked at the industry, in

1991. Insurance regulators liquidated two of those carriers, Farwest American and American Sun. The others voluntarily decided that long-term care insurance was not for them. One of those was Aetna, hardly a fly-by-night in the insurance industry.

"Companies are getting into this business as a sideline," says Irving Levit, president of Penn Treaty. "As time goes on, they find that all that glitters is not gold." Yet a gold rush continues, as companies, big and little, try to mine profits in the tricky field of long-term care insurance.

Carriers disappointed with their profits may stop selling new policies but continue to service and pay claims on the ones they have already sold. Or they may find another company to take over their coverage. When a policy is transferred in that manner, the policyholder may end up with a company even less financially secure than the old one.

"Companies are getting into this business as a sideline. As time goes on, they find that all that glitters is not gold."

The same thing can happen when carriers become insolvent. Before resorting to other measures, insurance departments may look for a new company to buy the defunct carrier's policies. The Oregon Insurance Department, for example, arranged for Universe Life to assume the long-term care policies of Farwest American. Farwest American's policyholders probably had never heard of Universe Life, let alone known anything of its financial condition. For many years, A.M. Best gave Universe Life, which was then primarily a life insurer, a B rating. In 1990, Best gave it no rating, pending an evaluation of how well it performed as a health insurance carrier.

ONE SAFETY NET

Policyholders of an insolvent company also may find their coverage provided by their state's life and health guaranty fund. When an insolvency occurs, all the carriers writing insurance in the state must chip in; the amount varies with how much business they do there. Fund administrators then use that money to pay policyholders' claims.

Although states created the guaranty funds, the fund administrators are not state agents and are not part of state insurance departments. The states themselves do not guarantee anyone's insurance coverage. During their sales pitches, agents are legally forbidden to mention the existence of the guaranty funds, which is probably just as well: When our reporter questioned agents about the funds, she found that they were unable to explain them correctly. One told our reporter that the state of Florida ultimately guaranteed all the policies—no need to worry.

There may indeed be need to worry. A guaranty fund that takes over a policy may cancel that policy if it is not guaranteed renewable. (Long-term care policies sold today are guaranteed renewable, but many earlier versions were not.) Even if their coverage is not canceled, policyholders may face serious delays in getting their claims paid. "The [guaranty] association may not know who the policyholders are," says Eden Sarfaty, president of the National Organization of Life and Health Insurance Guaranty Associations. "Records are poor. That's often the case with an insolvent company."

Most associations will guarantee only $100,000 of benefits for long-term care insurance. So a nursing-home stay that lasts several years may not be covered in full. The associations do not cover policies issued by fraternal organizations or by special trusts employers set up to provide health coverage. In most states they do *not* cover Blue Cross and Blue Shield plans. (And these days, the financial stability of Blue Cross organizations is a concern.)

Most associations cover only their own state residents if a company in that state becomes insolvent. Policyholders in other states must look to their state's guaranty fund for redress. In most cases, the funds will pay only if the insurance company was licensed to sell in that state—a potential problem for people who move to another state after buying a policy.

ADVICE TO CONSUMERS: SHOULD YOU BUY?

You have to be a bit of a gambler to buy a long-term care policy. Buyers must be willing to live with considerable uncertainty concerning rates, coverage, and even the insurance company's financial stability. Long-term care insurance is still a relatively new product, with many bugs to be worked out.

Before you think about buying a policy, consider both your income and your future assets. Ask yourself whether you will be able to afford the premium out of the income you are likely to have at the age of

70 or 75. For most retirees, the answer will be no. The average annual per capita income for someone age 65 is only about $17,000. If 65-year-olds of average income were to buy a good policy from a reputable company, they would spend more than $2,000 each year for coverage, or 12 percent of their income. Add to that another $1,000 or so for Medicare-supplement coverage, and decent protection comes to more than $3,000 a year, or $6,000 for a couple.

If your income is high enough to afford the premium, consider that the purpose of nursing-home insurance is as much to protect your savings and investments for your heirs as to buy space in a nursing home. If you are willing to use your savings to buy that space until your money runs out, Medicaid may pick up the costs once you are broke. But don't throw yourself lightly on your state's tender mercies. Many nursing homes dislike taking patients who are on Medicaid, because its reimbursement levels are low. If you depend on Medicaid, you may not be able to get into a nursing home of your choice.

Even if you buy long-term care insurance, you will, with many policies, still have a large out-of-pocket expense. If a 65-year-old is confined to a nursing home in the year 2010 and stays four years, the cost will exceed $317,000. A typical policy that pays $80 a day with no inflation protection would cover only $116,800, leaving $200,000 of uncovered expenses.

WHAT TO LOOK FOR

We recommend that consumers who want to take a chance on long-term care insurance buy a comprehensive policy that pays for both nursing-home care and home care. The latter may be built into the policy or sold as a rider. Choose home-care benefits that cover a wide range of services with the fewest restrictions.

Home-care-only policies have their appeal. Most people would rather stay at home than spend their last days in a nursing facility. However, if they become frail, they may eventually need nursing-home care anyway. When that time comes, a home-care only policy will be of little help in meeting expenses.

Good policies are expensive. We caution against buying a policy only because the premium is afford-able. It may offer inferior coverage, and its premiums may increase when you can least afford to pay more. Inflation protection is a must in our view, especially for anyone who buys the policy at a relatively young age. But many companies' inflation options are poor to mediocre. If you buy a policy, keep it. Do not switch plans just because an agent comes knocking at your door claiming to have a better one. Most policies do not have nonforfeiture benefits—you could lose your entire equity in the policy if you do switch.

If you already own a policy, we recommend that you keep it and buy additional coverage from your insurer if you feel your current policy is inadequate. If you own a policy that's very restrictive, you should weigh the likelihood of collecting benefits against the higher premiums you will probably have to pay for a new, less restrictive policy, as well as the loss of equi-ty you may have built up. Unfortunately, only a few companies offer policyholders the option to buy bet-ter coverage without proving they are still insurable, and fewer still allow policyholders to upgrade their benefits at a price reflecting the age they were when they first bought the policy. That's a desirable feature, in our view.

A final suggestion: Try to pay your premiums through an automatic draft arrangement with your bank. That minimizes your chances of losing the policy if you forget to pay, or are physically unable to pay, your premiums.

GROUP POLICIES

You may be able to buy a long-term care policy for yourself or a parent through your employer. Should you? The answer depends on the specifics of your employer's coverage. Insurance companies offer employers a basic plan, but most employers select the menu of benefits, waiting periods, and lifetime maximums. They also decide whether to offer inflation protection and nonforfeiture benefits, two valuable provisions described earlier. The insurance carrier generally chooses the gatekeepers, which determine when someone is eligible for benefits, and the levels of coverage. Unlike other employee benefits, employers usually pay none of the premiums.

The group policies we examined in 1991 were very like the ones offered to individuals. Their gatekeepers can be as liberal or as strict as in individual policies. The major difference between the two types of policy is the availability of nonforfeiture benefits. Such benefits were more likely to be found as an option in group contracts than in individual policies.

Buying through an employer has a few advantages.

Other Groups:
What's in a Name?

Employers are not the only ones offering group long-term care insurance. A few insurers have created "association" groups to market what are essentially individual policies. The names are designed to make you believe you are joining an organization rather than enlisting in an insurance company's marketing campaign.

To provide the group with an organizational cover, the company will probably offer discounts for travel, eyeglasses, and other items similar to the types of discounts offered by more legitimate organizations. The "associations" also give agents a supposed stamp of approval to tout. Associations may also provide a way for companies to skirt state insurance laws. By filing a "group" policy in one state with lax regulation, companies automatically gain approval to sell their policies in several other states. Yet when it's time for rate increases, carriers do not have to submit those increases for multistate approval.

Legitimate associations may also offer long-term care policies to their members. Our advice is the same. Carefully check the policy for yourself. Just because an association, even a bona fide association, offers a policy, that does not mean it's a good one.

Insurance companies may not be as particular about the health of currently employed workers as they are about those applying for individual coverage. They may do little or no checking on an employee's medical history. Some carriers may, in fact, accept all employees who apply. So if you have a condition that makes you uninsurable for an individual policy, your company's long-term care insurance may be your only option. (Insurers do, however, carefully check the health of parents and spouses who apply for coverage.) Policies offered through employers also may be less expensive than comparable individual plans, partly because sales costs are lower, and insurers can give large groups a price break.

Younger workers, usually those under age 50, often can buy coverage through employers before they are eligible to buy individual policies. However, we caution against buying a policy at that age unless it provides both inflation protection and nonforfeiture benefits. Some plans may offer neither, a short-sighted option, in our view. If you buy a fixed benefit at, say, age 45, and it isn't adjusted for inflation, the benefit will be worth practically nothing 40 years later when you are most likely to need nursing-home care. If you decide to buy through your employer, be sure you can continue your coverage if you change employers or if the employer terminates the plan. Look for provisions that allow you to continue with the same benefits and at the same price as your group coverage. If you do not find them, think twice before buying.

Try to have premiums deducted from your monthly pension check once you retire. That will ensure that your policy stays in force, and you won't have to worry about it lapsing.

GUIDELINES

If you are offered a policy through your employer and want to compare it with an individual policy, look first at the gatekeepers and the coverage. If the group policy has restrictive gatekeepers and coverage, you might do better with an individual policy from the same insurer or from a different one.

The conventional advice to buy from a company rated A or A+ by A.M. Best is no longer fool-proof. One safeguard is to buy from a carrier that has reinsured its long-term care policies; that is, it has paid another carrier to assume some of the risk. However, as part of *Consumer Reports'* 1991 survey, when we asked carriers whether they reinsured, many refused to tell us.

There's no way to judge whether an insurance company trying to sell you a long-term care policy is in the business for the long haul or the quick buck. Aside from avoiding companies that are already in trouble, there's little shoppers can do to assure themselves that the company they pick today will be at their side tomorrow.

People considering long-term care insurance should check with their state's insurance department to see whether their state has a guaranty fund to take care of policyholders of insolvent companies. And if such a fund exists, shoppers should also inquire whether it would cover them even if they bought from an out-of-state company.

If you find that this report leaves you with miser-

191

able alternatives, that's because long-term care policies are not good enough. To make them better, state regulators or Congress must require companies to include mandatory inflation and nonforfeiture protection and place some reasonable limits on how much rates can increase. Ideally, insurance companies would also be required to offer only a limited number of standardized policies so that consumers could readily compare them. Such improvements would lead to higher premiums. And therein lies the contradiction of long-term care insurance. For the coverage to do a proper job of paying nursing expenses for the elderly, it will almost certainly have to cost more. And the more it costs, the fewer the people who will be able to afford it.

THE SEARCH FOR A BETTER WAY

6
ALTERNATIVE SYSTEMS: CANADA, HAWAII, MINNESOTA

"One option Canadians are not considering is a move back to a system like the one we have in the United States."

More than 30 years ago, Canada enacted a program to bring health care within reach of all its citizens. By 1971, Canada's provincial governments were paying the medical bills for everyone in Canada, and few people outside Canada were paying much attention.

As the U.S. health care system began to creak and groan under the weight of its runaway costs, and as its inability to serve every citizen became increasingly apparent, Americans started to look seriously at Canada's health care system as a model for reform. At the same time, Canada's system started to come under concerted attack from those special-interest groups—health-insurance companies, medical associations, and hospitals—that profit most from the present U.S. *non*system of health care. This chapter examines the strengths and weaknesses of the Canadian system and evaluates the criticisms leveled against it.

It also looks at two states, Hawaii and Minnesota, which have experimented with other ways of reforming and broadening the health care system.

Finally, it will set forth Consumers Union's own proposal for a U.S. health care system that meets three important criteria: universality, affordability, and high quality.

HOW THE CANADIAN SYSTEM WORKS

Contrary to what some in the U.S. health care industry would have you believe, Canada does not have "socialized medicine." Medicare, as Canada's health care system is called, is simply a social insurance plan, much like the U.S. Social Security and Medicare systems for older Americans. Canada's doctors do *not* work on salary for the government.

Canadians pay for health care through a variety of federal and provincial taxes, just as Americans pay for Social Security and Medicare through payroll taxes. The government of each province pays the medical bills for its citizens. Because the government is the primary payer of medical bills, Canada's system is referred to as a "single-payer" arrangement. Benefits vary somewhat among the provinces, but most cover, in addition to medical and hospital care, long-term care, mental-health services, and prescription drugs for people over 65. Private insurance exists only for those services the provincial plans do not cover.

Although each province runs its own insurance program as it sees fit, all are guided by the five principles of the Canada Health Act.

1. *Universality*: Everyone in the nation is covered.
2. *Portability*: People can move from province to province and from job to job (or onto the unemployment rolls) and still retain their health coverage.
3. *Accessibility*: Everyone has access to the system's health care providers.
4. *Comprehensiveness*: Provincial plans cover all medically necessary treatment.
5. *Public administration*: The system is publicly run and publicly accountable.

The role of doctors in the Canadian system is little understood in the United States and is frequently distorted by the foes of a single-payer system. For example, in announcing his plan for health reform last winter, President Bush declared: "We don't need to put government between patients and their doctors and create another wasteful federal bureaucracy." Nor should the government tell doctors how to practice medicine, other opponents of Canadian-style health care often add.

Canada's health care system does neither. "In the U.S., there's a myth that Canadians have an awful government bureaucracy that tells doctors how to practice medicine," says Dr. Michael Rachlis, a Toronto physician and health-policy consultant. "There's much more interference from third parties [such as insurance companies and utilization review firms] in the U.S. than from the government in Canada."

"In the U.S., there's a myth that Canadians have an awful government bureaucracy that tells doctors how to practice medicine."

Canada's physicians practice in their own offices and work for themselves, just as most U.S. doctors do. The main difference: Canadian doctors may not charge whatever they wish. Their fees are set according to a schedule negotiated by each provincial medical association with its province's ministry of health. Canadian doctors cannot engage in the common American practice of "balance billing"—billing the patient the difference between what an insurer will pay and what the doctor wishes to charge.

The negotiation process has managed to keep fee inflation in Canada at least modestly in check. Fees tend to be much lower than those commanded by American doctors for the same service. In British

Columbia, for example, doctors receive about $349 to remove a gallbladder; in Manitoba, $354; and in Ontario, $348 (all figures are in U.S. dollars). But in New York City, the customary fee paid by insurance carriers averages about $2,700; in Buffalo, New York, $945.

Despite the lower fees, physicians in Canada, like those in the United States, enjoy high incomes. In British Columbia, the average payment (before overhead) made by the health ministry to cardiologists last year was $290,500; to ophthalmologists, $240,500; to dermatologists, $200,500; and to general practitioners, $128,000.

Canadians, like U.S. citizens, can select any doctor they like. Those doctors bill the provincial insurance plans directly and are usually paid within two to four weeks. For patients, there are no bills, claim forms, out-of-pocket costs, or waits for reimbursement from insurance carriers, all common complaints here.

Roughly half of all Canadian physicians are family practitioners (compared to 13 percent here), and Canadians go to them for treatment that Americans might seek from costlier specialists. Most Canadians, for instance, take their children to family practitioners instead of to pediatricians for common childhood illnesses. Most children see pediatricians only for serious problems. The provinces encourage people who need a specialist's care to obtain a referral from a family doctor, much the way HMOs and other managed-care plans do in the United States. If a specialist sees a patient who has not obtained a referral, that specialist can bill the government only the fee that would ordinarily have been paid to a general practitioner. But those rules, aimed at controlling costs by preventing the overuse of high-priced specialists, do not always have their intended effect. If a patient shows up at a specialist's office without a referral, the specialist need only call the family practitioner, obtain a referral number, and bill the government the higher fee.

THE DRAWBACKS—REAL AND SUPPOSED

Many of Canada's family doctors are only too glad to send any complicated or time-consuming case to a specialist, as the rules permit, so that they can see more patients and earn more fees. The increased use of medical services is a major reason costs are escalating there as they are here. Canada's rising health care costs are, of course, a favorite target of U.S. critics.

Much has been made of the fact that Canadian hospitals have reduced their number of beds in recent months. The implication is that the Canadian health care system is collapsing and that Canadians now suffer from insufficient hospital facilities. Actually, Canada has too many hospital beds, which is also the case here. Hospitals proliferated in both countries during the last two decades. Money flowed freely, building new hospitals was good politics, and the public as well as the government came to believe that another hospital bed meant better health care.

As health care costs in Canada rise, the provinces are being forced to rethink how best to spend their

health dollars. Most bed closings stem from deliber-
ate government strategies to eliminate waste and
duplication of services. In Toronto, for example,
where a total of 2,200 beds have been permanently
closed, the city's 45 hospitals still have 1,000 beds
empty on any given day.

Provincial governments can implement such cost-
cutting measures because they control how much
money a hospital receives. Every year they negotiate
a "global budget" with each hospital in the province.
That budget includes money to cover operating costs,
increases for inflation and greater utilization, and any
special services the ministry wants the hospital to
offer. The global budgets set by the provincial governments comprise about 95 percent of a hospital's
total funds. Any other money must come from
fundraising and investment earnings. Within the
global budgets, hospitals are free to move money
around. If, say, a hospital finds the costs of running
the emergency room are lower than expected, it can
redirect some of the money to increase the number
of cataract surgeries, if it chooses to. Canadian hospitals, however, are not allowed to run deficits.

Long waits for low-tech care? Perhaps the
most frequently heard charge against the Canadian
system is that it rations care and that people do not
get the treatment they need. *The New York Times* told
readers of its editorial page last November that, as a
result of "rationing," Canadian women "must wait
months for a simple Pap smear."

In reality, women in Canada routinely have Pap

smears done by their family doctors, who perform them the same way U.S. doctors do. Canada's ambassador to the United States traced the tale of Pap smear waits to a brief delay in laboratory processing in Newfoundland some years ago—a problem long since corrected.

Canadian men and women routinely have general surgery, diagnostic ultrasound, X-rays, thyroid tests, amniocentesis, electrocardiograms, and hundreds of other procedures and treatments without delay. But Canadians may not have immediate access to the latest technological innovations, such as lithotripters (machines that crush kidney stones with sound waves) and magnetic resonance imagers (MRIs), or to such surgical procedures as a coronary-artery bypass or hip replacement. Someone who pulls a knee muscle playing soccer is unlikely to get an MRI scan the day after the accident. And those who want bypass surgery to relieve angina symptoms will not be wheeled into the operating room right away. However, anyone requiring emergency care gets it immediately.

Because provincial governments control hospital budgets, they also control the introduction and use of technology. In some cases, they have kept a tight lid on that technology to restrain the high costs associated with excessive, inappropriate, or duplicative use. Hospitals denied some piece of equipment by the provincial health ministry are free to buy it with money raised from private contributions, but they cannot look to the ministry for funds to operate it. In Winnipeg, Manitoba, for example, Seven Oaks Hospital purchased a computerized tomography (CT) scanner with its own funds and is already operating it. The Ministry of Health maintains that the province does not need this CT scanner, that the six scanners already available at other provincial hospitals are enough to serve the province's needs. The ministry has hinted that it may not cover the $1-million operating and depreciation expenses for the machine.

The ministry has taken a hard line on MRIs as well. The province has one, and the hospital operating it must follow strict guidelines in deciding when it should be used. The province probably could use another MRI machine, says Dr. Cam Mustard, an assistant professor of community health sciences at the University of Manitoba. But, he adds, "it's not such a scarce resource that people are coming to harm because they can't get on it. Doctors are very satisfied with the quality of service, and the waiting times are not seen as obstructing their ability to care for patients."

"The alternative [to having such waiting times]," says Dr. Charles Wright, a vice president for medicine at Vancouver General Hospital, "is to have a grossly overbuilt system, as in the U.S. If you build for the peaks, you have a hell of a lot of wasted resources."

The published figures on the number of Canadians on waiting lists probably exaggerate the actual delays in receiving care. For the most part, doctors manage the lists, putting people on one or more of them as they deem appropriate. Sometimes doctors put a patient on a list to give him or her hope when a condition is actually hopeless. Sometimes they do so just in case a patient's condition should worsen and a procedure not now necessary becomes necessary. Queues shift constantly, as those needing care immediately move ahead of those whose conditions are less serious. Sometimes queues develop and then disappear. At Wellesley Hospital in Toronto, for example, kidney patients once faced a three-month wait for lithotripsy. Now there is virtually no wait, and the machine does not always run at capacity.

When St. Boniface Hospital in Winnipeg investigated its waiting list of 143 people for cardiac angiography, a radiological examination of the arteries surrounding the heart, it found that only 56 people were really candidates for the procedure. Some did not need it, some did not want it, and some had already had the procedure done at another hospital. One doctor was accused of packing the list for his own political reasons.

In 1991, in British Columbia, a Royal Commission on health care investigated all the well-publicized cases of people who claimed to have been harmed by delays in the queue for heart surgery. "When we tracked them down, almost all of the cases crumbled," says Appeals Court Justice Peter Seaton, who chaired the commission.

That finding has scarcely stopped opponents of Canadian-style health care from citing waiting lists in British Columbia as evidence that the system is grinding to a halt. "A waiting list of 700 to 800 people for heart surgery is not uncommon," a vice-president of the National Center for Public Policy Research, a conservative think-tank, wrote in a 1992 *New York Times* column.

A waiting list of that length did exist, but only for a short time. When researchers looked into it, they found that two-thirds of the people on the list were waiting not for the procedure, but for three particular surgeons.

When waiting lists have grown too long, provincial governments have in some instances offered patients the option of going to the United States for treatment. The British Columbia Ministry of Health, for example, contracted with hospitals in Seattle to provide 200 heart surgeries. It took more than a year before Canadians filled all 200 slots, raising the question of whether the delays were indeed life-threatening.

Critics like to portray the availability of treatment in the United States as a safety valve for Canadians. However, that says as much about the overcapacity of the American system as it does about poor planning on the part of Canada. The British Columbia Health Ministry received many calls from U.S. hospitals eagerly soliciting its heart-surgery business.

Unavailable operations? When he was running for the Democratic presidential nomination, former Senator Paul Tsongas said that if he had lived in Canada, he would be dead by now. The procedure that arrested his cancer, Tsongas said, was not available there. In fact, the procedure that saved Tsongas's life, autologous bone-marrow transplantation, was available in Canada in 1986 when Tsongas had his operation. Indeed, the pioneering research that led to bone-marrow transplants took place at a Toronto hospital 30 years ago.

In making his charge, Tsongas joined the long list of critics of the Canadian health care system who contend that it denies its citizens appropriate care. The National Center for Public Policy Research, for example, has asserted that "Canadians do not have enough surgery, at least not enough of the surgery they need the most." And Newt Gingrich, the Republican whip in the House of Representatives, has contended that "it is illegal in Canada to get a whole series of operations."

If anything, Canadians are probably getting too much care, just as Americans are. A report prepared for the Conference of Deputy Ministers of Health last year found that a "nontrivial" amount of the medical services Canadians receive are ineffective and inappropriate. The report blamed fee-for-service reimbursements to doctors for much of the problem. The same criticism applies to the United States, as we detailed in Chapter 1.

Surgery rates for some procedures are actually higher in Canada than elsewhere. Canada is a world leader in the number of gallbladder surgeries and is second only to the United States in heart-bypass operations. Each year, the French perform 15 to 20 bypass surgeries per 100,000 people; the British, 20 to 30; the Canadians, 50; and the Americans, about 100.

Higher mortality? In health care reform proposals put forward earlier this year, the Bush Administration asserted that "postoperative mortality is 44 percent higher in Canada than in the U.S. for high-risk procedures, including heart surgery." Dr. Leslie Roos, a professor of community health sciences at the University of Manitoba and one of the authors of the study to which the Administration referred, told Consumers Union that the statement "seriously distorts our overall findings." For one thing, the study compared only Manitoba and New England, not Canada and the United States. For another, it compared a number of low-risk and moderate-risk procedures, and only two that were high-risk (namely, repair of hip fracture and concurrent valve replacement with bypass, one kind of heart surgery). The study showed that for the low- and moderate-risk procedures, the number of people who died shortly after surgery was similar in the two regions. The mortality rates for hip-fracture repair in New England were lower than in Manitoba, primarily because many Manitoba patients had to be transported long distances from remote, northern parts of the province. Roos told us that later research is showing Manitoba's heart-surgery results "to be fully comparable with those of the leading American centers." He added that three-year survival rates for cardiovascular surgery are better in Manitoba than they are in the United States.

HOW COSTS COMPARE

As noted, opponents of a single-payer system like to claim that health care costs are rising faster in Canada than in the United States. A study by the Health Insurance Association of America (HIAA), the insurance companies' trade organization, reported that per capita spending in the United States rose, on average, 4.38 percent per year from 1967 to 1987, compared with 4.58 percent in Canada. But Canada's single-payer system was not completely in place until 1971. Although other researchers have refuted the HIAA's findings, the numbers live on in propaganda against the Canadian system.

Health care costs *are* lower in Canada than here, whether measured by per capita spending or as a percentage of gross national product. In 1989, the United States spent $2,450 per person on health care, while Canada spent $1,800. In 1990, the United States spent 12.2 percent of its GNP on health care; Canada spent 9.5 percent.

Before Canada fully implemented its Medicare system in 1971, both it and the United States were spending comparable amounts of their respective GNPs on health care. But as Canada's system of universal coverage took hold in all the provinces, spending by the two countries sharply diverged.

Canadian researchers believe that 25 to 35 percent of the difference may be due to Canada's controls on hospitals. One study found that in the early 1980s, for instance, the United States spent as much as 50 percent more per person on hospital services, even though Canadians stayed in the hospital longer, on average. But perhaps the most striking differences are in administrative costs. In 1987, researchers have estimated, the United States spent between 19 and 24 percent of its health care dollars on administrative expenses; Canada spent between 8 and 11 percent.

LONG-TERM CARE IN CANADA

All Canadians are eligible for government-paid long-term care, no matter how high their incomes or how much money they have in the bank. They are not forced to "spend down" their assets or impoverish themselves before the government will pay for their care, as many Americans are (see Chapter 5).

Canadians who use long-term care services must pay a modest amount for them, currently between $17 and $21 a day. In British Columbia, for instance, residents in long-term care facilities pay about $19 toward the typical $67 daily charge for nursing-home care. The Ministry of Health pays the rest. That payment is adjusted periodically, based on changes in the cost of living and in government-financed pensions.

If someone also receives welfare or old-age assistance from the government, the government deducts the amount it pays toward nursing-home care from those payments. But a person in that situation is still left with more disposable income than nursing-home residents in the United States who receive Medicaid benefits. In Canada, patients can keep between $84 and $143 each month for incidental expenses. A nursing-home resident in New York City who receives Medicaid can keep only $50.

Provinces differ in the long-term care services they provide and in how people gain access to them. British Columbia and Manitoba are the most advanced, allowing residents to enter their long-term care systems through a "single entry." If people in British Columbia, for example, need long-term care,

Canadian Health Care Politics

Much of the ammunition fired by U.S. critics at the Canadian system has inadvertently been supplied by the Canadians themselves in internal political skirmishes. When it comes time to negotiate fees or new budgets, doctors and other providers there often assert that the Canadian system is underfunded.

Providers make waiting lists a political issue or put their case before the public by writing letters and running advertisements that take their health care system to task. This spring, a Manitoba Medical Association newsletter featured an open letter to the minister of health; the headline read: "Rationing Eye Surgery Impairs Patients' Quality of Life, MMA President Tells Minister." The publication also ran letters from a doctor and a patient's relative pleading for more money for hip-replacement surgery. The British Columbia Medical Association ran newspaper ads warning of the harm that could come from placing a cap on the fees earned by its highest-paid members, such as ophthalmologists, dermatologists, and cardiologists; the cap was a strategy the ministry was pursuing to reduce health care expenditures.

Conflicts between Canada's health care providers

and the government, however, are often overblown in the United States. Not long ago, Dr. Gur S. Singh, then president of the British Columbia Medical Association, sent a letter to provincial newspapers arguing that Americans should keep their system basically unchanged. Singh said he wanted the United States to "continue to provide the necessary safety valve to an overly restrictive Canadian system which will only get worse as further bureaucratic controls are adopted." The president of the Health Insurance Association of America, Carl Schramm, in testimony to the U.S. Senate, quoted from Singh's letter. At the end of the letter, Singh did say that the Canadian system was "one of the best, and perhaps it still is the best health care system in the world." However, that point did not make it into Schramm's testimony.

An astute Canadian observer would have known that Singh's letter was simply a "piece of negotiating rhetoric intended to bat the Minister [of Health] over the head," Dr. Hedy Fry, Singh's predecessor at the medical group, informed us: "That letter was for public consumption in B.C."

they or their families contact one of the Health Ministry's 90 offices. The ministry then dispatches case managers who direct patients to appropriate services, such as medical treatment, home care, day-care centers, or nursing-home care. In the United States, people needing long-term care have no one entry point. They must first get a doctor to certify that they need nursing-home care and then shop around for a facility willing to take them.

The ministry also has created 15 quick-response teams that act when an older person seeks treatment in a hospital emergency room. These teams identify people who can be helped with early intervention, such as patients who have broken hips. The idea is to get them the right kind of treatment immediately, rather than let them languish in costly hospital rooms.

Other provinces are beginning to follow the lead of Manitoba and British Columbia in establishing a single-entry system for their citizens' long-term care. Each province is also trying to move long-term patients who do not need to be hospitalized out of hospitals and into less expensive community and home-care settings. The single-payer system is well suited for that task, since it allows health ministries to decide where to direct their money. In British Columbia, for example, the ministry has increased by 9 percent the number of hours of home care it will pay for, while increasing the number of nursing-home beds only by about 2 percent. "You can create incentives to direct people to community-based services," says Paul Pallan, an assistant deputy minister in the province's Ministry of Health.

A HEALTHY, IF IMPERFECT, SYSTEM

The Canadian health care system, like every health care system in the world, has problems, though they are not of the scary sort usually cited by U.S. critics. There is a more-than-adequate supply of doctors in Canada, but there is a shortage of physicians in the remote, northern areas of the country, where few want to practice. The United States has the same problem, of course; few doctors care to practice in rural or poverty-stricken areas.

"You can create incentives to direct people to community-based services."

Even though Canada has a greater proportion of family doctors than we do, medical school incentives have steered doctors-in-training to specialties that command higher fees and result in higher costs to the system. (In Chapter 1, we note the same phenomenon in the United States.) A report presented to Canada's deputy ministers of health last year blamed at least part of this trend on the bad example of the United States, where 87 percent of all physicians are specialists and only one-third or less practice so-called primary care.

A more fundamental flaw is that, through the years, provincial governments have acted more like check-writers than health care managers. As in the United States, hospitals and doctors often received generous

213

increases simply by asking for them. In Ontario, for instance, hospital spending has increased 10 percent or more each year for the last 10 years. But that is changing. This year Ontario hospitals are getting just a 1 percent increase in their global budgets, and the ministry is redirecting money to other types of health care.

Canadian patients also may have stayed in hospitals longer than was necessary. In 1989, the average length of stay was 10.5 days, compared to 7.2 days here. In Canada, patients are still entering hospitals a day or two before their surgeries for preoperative workups, a practice that U.S. utilization firms are rapidly putting an end to.

Since 1984, health care spending by the provinces has increased 80 percent, to about $44 billion. At the same time, the economy that funds that spending has grown less than 20 percent. The Canadian federal government, which once provided about 50 percent of the funding for the provincial health budgets, now supplies only about 35 percent. Eventually it may leave the funding solely to the provinces. Pushed by rising costs and by pressures on funding, the provinces are redirecting money and starting programs to make better use of their dollars. "We're afraid we're going to lose our system if we don't change it," says Lin Grist, a special assistant to Ontario's Minister of Health. "It's really quite precious to us."

The United States faces similar problems, but Canada is in a better position to solve them. For one thing, it long ago answered the question of whether everyone in the country is entitled to health care—a question the United States seems incapable of actively resolving. For another, Canada's single-payer system is better suited to the task of redeploying resources as needed. It can decide where to spend its budget for the good of all citizens.

In the United States, the rhetoric of the day is to contain costs. But few, if any, doctors or other providers embrace limits on their own incomes. And no single payer has enough influence to impose the controls necessary to squeeze the billions of dollars of waste out of the system.

One option Canadians are *not* considering is a move back to a system like the one we have. Of the 1,503 people who testified before the British Columbia Royal Commission in its hearings on health reform, only one favored adopting the American way of paying for health care. Canadians like their health care system and expect their government to fix its current problems. But a government that tried to tinker with the basic principles of the Canada Health Act would be a government out of power very soon.

U.S. INSURERS ON THE ATTACK

The popularity of the Canadian system among Canadians has not prevented the U.S. insurance industry, among others who profit from our current system, from badmouthing it in an organized public relations campaign. Two years ago, Carl Schramm, president of the Health Insurance Association of America

(HIAA), told Consumers Union that the greatest strength of his organization was "educational" lobbying. "We produce lots of research bulletins that are classy little numbers," Schramm said.

At least one of those classy little numbers, attacking the Canadian health care system, has reached far and wide. A few years ago, as we noted earlier in the chapter, the HIAA compared the amounts that Canada and the United States spent on health care, per capita, and found that from 1967 to 1987 Canada's

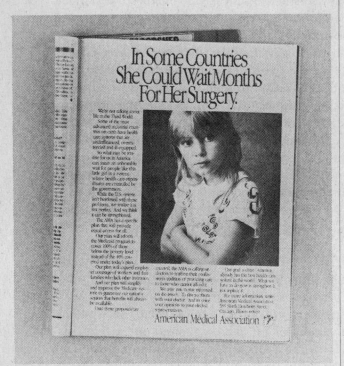

To counteract positive portrayals of universal health insurance in Canada and elsewhere, the American Medical Association ran a national ad campaign in 1989.

growth rate was slightly higher: 4.58 percent compared to 4.38 percent in the United States. From that statistic, it concluded that Canada has done no better than we have in controlling the escalation of health care costs.

Other researchers, including an American, a Canadian, and an Australian, refuted the HIAA's claim, pointing out that the trade association had chosen a 20-year period beginning four years before all the provinces had fully phased in universal health insurance. When those years are removed from the analysis, the data show that Canada's per capita health care spending actually grew more slowly than that of the United States. And when researchers extended the period of comparison two more years, to 1989, they found that real growth in costs (which takes inflation into account) had actually declined in Canada after 1987, while they had continued to increase here.

Even more persuasive is a comparison of how much of its gross national product each country spends on health care. In 1971, the year Canada fully implemented its system, both it and the United States spent 7.4 percent of their respective GNPs on health care. By 1989, Canada was spending 8.9 percent, compared to our 11.6 percent. That 2.7-percent difference in share of GNP devoted to health care represents about $125 billion that the United States could have put to other uses.

Edward Neuschler, director of policy development and research for the HIAA, conceded to Consumers Union that "the GNP comparison is a valid one to make. To the Canadians' credit, they certainly do spend less." Yet it's the HIAA's selective statistics that turn up, often in disguised form, when critics attack Canada's single-payer system.

Blue Cross/Blue Shield of Missouri paid for an eight-page advertising supplement that appeared in the spring of 1992 in the *St. Louis Post Dispatch* and 14 other Missouri newspapers and periodicals. Residents of Hannibal, Jefferson City, Poplar Bluff, and Springfield were told that per capita spending on health care increased more slowly in the United States than in Canada from 1967 to 1987. Blue Cross/Blue Shield documented that claim in a footnote citing a magazine called *Business & Health*, rather than the HIAA. *Business & Health* is a publication prepared "in consultation with" the Washington Business Group on Health, an organization whose members are large corporations. The *Business & Health* report attributed its figures to a study done by the National Center for Policy Analysis.

"To the Canadians' credit, they certainly do spend less."

The National Center for Policy Analysis is a conservative, Dallas-based think-tank whose board of directors includes representatives of corporations such as Southland, ARCO, and Golden Rule Insurance. Golden Rule, based in Indianapolis, is a large seller of individual health and Medicare-supplement policies. The company would stand to lose much of its business if the nation adopted a single-payer system.

Since 1988, the National Center for Policy Analysis has produced 59 reports and two books on a range of topics. Its study, "Twenty Myths About National Health Insurance," released in December 1991, appears to be the source *Business & Health* used in its story. Myth No. 1, according to the Center's report, is that "countries with national health insurance have been more successful than the U.S. in controlling health care costs." It contradicts the "myth" by referring to the disputed findings of the HIAA study.

THE NEWEST ANTI-CANADA CAMPAIGN

Now, the results of a new HIAA study called "Timely Attitudes" are beginning to make the rounds. Based on telephone polling, the report summarizes what voters think about a number of health issues and proposals for reform.

The report's "executive summary" contends that the public is *not* "eager to scrap our current health insurance system and embrace a Canadian-style system." The report itself, however, shows that 60 percent of respondents would favor such a system. Then, the report says, "support for the Canadian system declined once the trade-offs (cost, delays, less focus on new technologies) were presented"—in other words, once the usual distortions of Canada's system were accepted as fact.

Based on the new study, the HIAA is running an ad campaign on Washington, D.C., television stations and in such influential publications as *Congressional*

Quarterly, National Journal, The New Republic, and *Roll Call.* The ads invite readers to write for more information about the survey.

If the American people are indeed content with the U.S. health care system, that might in itself be testimony to the power of the HIAA's misinformation campaign. However, other polls dispute the HIAA view of public opinion. A 1990 *Los Angeles Times* poll found that 66 percent of Americans would prefer the Canadian health care system to their own. That almost replicated a 1988 Louis Harris poll, which found that 61 percent of Americans preferred the Canadian system—a number that almost precisely matches the HIAA's own 60-percent figure.

CANADIAN VS. U.S. HEALTH CARE: CASE STUDIES

How does the Canadian system look to those for whom it was designed, the patients? To find out, *Consumer Reports* located U.S. and Canadian families and individuals with roughly the same health situations and compared their experiences seeking, getting, and paying for medical care.

FAMILIES WITH MANY NEEDS

United States: Afraid to use the insurance they have. Randy Sadler owns a tile business in Kernersville, North Carolina. His wife, Denise, works part-time as a field representative for the U.S. Census Bureau. Their two boys, Brent, age

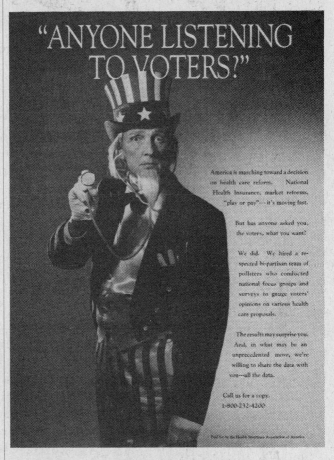

Ads like this one appear in "opinion leader" magazines, urging readers to send for the HIAA report.

9, and Ben, age 7, have the usual childhood illnesses. Ben, however, also has severe allergies and often has pneumonia and other complications. Brent has symptoms of allergies, but a doctor has never diagnosed them. Denise gets migraine headaches and suffers from depression. Randy is healthy.

221

Until recently, the Sadlers had no health insurance. Denise works too few hours for the federal government to qualify for her employer's coverage, and Randy, being self-employed, had no insurance. The family earns roughly the U.S. median income of about $35,000 a year. Realizing how risky it is to be without insurance, the family bought two policies from American Republic: one for Randy, with a $1,000 deductible, and one for Denise and the boys, who each must satisfy a $500 deductible every year. The monthly premiums total $227.

A sales brochure promised a 5 percent premium reduction if, during any year, no family members covered by the policy filed a claim. However, if someone later submits a claim, the reduction is wiped out, and the premium reverts to what it would have been. The promise of lower premiums is a potent inducement to keep the Sadlers from filing claims. "I still feel like we have no insurance," says Denise.

They might as well not have. Ben, the child who is frequently ill, has no coverage for the very conditions that make him sick, a common feature of commercial U.S. health insurance (as explained in Chapter 2). American Republic has "waivered" his coverage for allergies, except for acute reactions that require hospitalization. It has also waivered his coverage for ear disorders and for diseases of his tonsils and adenoids. For Denise, the company has waivered treatment for allergies, but not for migraines or depression.

At the time she applied for coverage, Denise had not sought treatment for depression. She put off seeing a doctor and delayed a gynecological checkup because she knew insurance carriers disapproved of applicants who had recently been to the doctor.

Ben has had two operations to put tubes in his ears, which the family has paid for little by little. The Sadlers have just paid off the surgery center and the doctor who performed Ben's latest ear surgery two years ago; they still owe the anesthesiologist $173. But bills for Ben's care—biweekly allergy shots, medicines for recurring ear infections, doctor visits—are mounting again. And, of course, their insurance policy is of no help.

The family typically spends $100 to $200 a month on medical care and prescription drugs, in addition to their health insurance premiums. Last November, Brent was hospitalized for what doctors thought was spinal meningitis, and Denise sprained her knee playing ball with the boys. That month, their medical bills came to $1,500.

Paying for prescription drugs is a problem, but one that their physicians are solving for good or ill. Their doctors, knowing the family's precarious financial situation, freely hand out samples of medications that pharmaceutical companies have given them. By giving doctors and patients free samples, the drug companies hope to win converts to their products. Doctors have given Denise free samples of Prozac, an antidepressant. The drug ordinarily costs $91 a month if Denise takes one pill a day and twice that if she takes two. Since the beginning of the year, her doctor has given her about $300 worth of Prozac capsules. She has spent another $200 of her own money to buy more of the drug.

Canada: High medical needs, generous coverage. Like the Sadlers, the Deveys of Burlington, Ontario, have relied heavily upon medical services lately. Linda, 46, has had a number of gynecological procedures, and she also has severe allergies. Her sons, Philip, age 18, and Murray, age 12, have similar allergies. Their father Robert, 51, suffers from recurring cysts on the cornea of one eye.

Robert is a teacher; Linda, a teacher's assistant. The family's gross income last year was about $60,000 in U.S. dollars. Of that, they paid about $14,600 in federal and provincial taxes. Some of those taxes go to fund the Ontario Health Insurance Plan, which pays most of the family's medical bills. The school district that employs Robert pays $600 a year for "extended health insurance" that pays for some of the medical treatment not covered by the province. The district also buys dental coverage for the family. That benefit costs the school district $700 a year. In Canada, about 25 percent of all health expenditures are either paid out of pocket or covered by private insurance.

The Deveys' allergies are so severe that conventional treatment by an allergist—an "average" dose of allergen extract to counteract the symptoms—is of no help. So they see a doctor of environmental medicine who, Linda says, does more extensive testing to arrive at a specific dose of extract that neutralizes their symptoms. The treatment helps, but Ontario's health plan pays only for visits to the doctor, not for the injections or the testing, which it considers experimental. The Deveys must look to their extended health coverage to pay for the injections, which cost about $1,100 last year. The Deveys themselves paid about $1,700 for testing and allergy treatments.

Their out-of-pocket expenses used to be higher. For a while, Mutual Life of Canada, the carrier that underwrites their extended health policy, refused to pay for the injections, also claiming that the treatment was experimental. Linda appealed the company's decision to Ontario's Human Rights Commission and won. That victory has reduced their expenses for the injections by half.

They have virtually no other medical expenses, however, since Ontario's plan takes care of just about everything else. Otherwise, "we'd be in the poorhouse," says Linda. In the last few years, she has had two operations to remove benign cysts in her ovaries and breast. Because of her allergies, she had to be in a special hospital room. The hospital care, she says, was "superb."

In February, Linda suffered a whiplash injury in an automobile accident. The Ontario health plan paid for her care in the emergency room, X-rays, and 10 visits to a physiotherapist. It covered part of the bill for three visits to a chiropractor, but nothing for a massage therapist she saw. The extended health policy picked up the remainder of the chiropractor's bills, and Linda paid $42 for the massage.

When Robert needed treatment for his eye, Ontario covered the five physician visits he required, and the extended health coverage paid for the $168 worth of antibiotics. When the boys need treatment for ear infections, they often use an "after-hours" clinic. Such facilities, staffed by medical professionals, are popping up all over Canada; the provinces pay for the care they deliver.

Doctors in Ontario are allowed to bill their patients small amounts—$5, $10, or $15—for such services as prescribing medication over the telephone, transferring medical records to another doctor, making appointments with specialists, and filling out immunization reports or health forms for children's camps and schools. The Deveys' doctor gives his patients the choice of paying an annual fee of $54 that takes care of all those services or paying as the need arises. The Deveys take their chances and pay only when they need the service.

CATASTROPHIC MEDICAL NEEDS

United States: Staying poor to obtain care. The Winslows of Lincolnville, Maine, are a young family with two children. Daughter Jessie, age 7, was born with bipolar disorder, which causes manic-depressive behavior; it is a rare condition in young children. Five-year-old Savannah has chronic ear infections, temporarily impairing her hearing and speech.

Deb, the children's mother, suffers from asthma, skin rashes, and migraine headaches. Tom, their father, is a healthy, self-employed carpenter. His gross income last year was about $21,000. The family's medical expenses, including health insurance premiums to Blue Cross/Blue Shield of Maine, eat up nearly 20 percent of that income.

Their Blue Cross policy, which costs about $3,200 a year, pays the usual 80 percent for doctors' charges and prescription drugs, but only $84 a day for hospital care. The local hospital charges $500 a day. The policy also limits benefits for mental illness. It pays just 50 percent of the cost of Jessie's weekly therapy, up to a lifetime maximum of $20,000. The Winslows figure they will have exhausted those benefits by the time Jessie is 12.

Deb quit her job as a bookkeeper to reduce the family's income enough so that Jessie would qualify for Medicaid, the federal–state program that covers medical bills for the poor. "We have to stay poor," Deb says. With Medicaid paying for some of Jessie's treatment, the Winslows hope their Blue Cross benefits will last longer.

Blue Cross recently increased the Winslows' monthly premium from $270 to $330, so they have applied for a cheaper policy. That policy, however, will pay for only 26 weeks of therapy for Jessie, instead of 52 . "We've kept the policy because we didn't feel it was fair for the state to pay for Jessie," says Deb. "But you have to feed your children, too."

The Winslows also have to stay poor to provide care for Savannah. She recently qualified for the Maine Health Program, a new state- and federally funded plan that covers medical bills for about 5,400 of Maine's poorest children. The Winslows pay a premium of $9.55 each month.

The paperwork for the multiple plans has put Deb's bookkeeping skills to the test. The Blue Cross subsidiary, Blue Alliance, that provides the family's major medical coverage must pay its share of the children's bills before Medicaid and the Maine Health Program kick in. The pharmacy that supplies Jessie's $200 worth of prescriptions each month must first bill Medicaid. Medicaid then sends the Winslows a form to mail Blue Alliance. Blue Alliance pays Medicaid 80 percent of the bill, and Medicaid then pays the pharmacy the amount it has received from Blue Alliance plus the portion it's obligated to cover. When Deb needs a prescription for herself, she pays the pharmacy, then must wait up to 12 weeks for reimbursement from the insurer, forcing the family to put off paying other bills.

Deb needs prescription-strength inhalers to prevent asthma attacks, but their $57 price tag makes them a luxury. "If I used them according to instructions, I'd have to buy them every month, so I use them only when I get an attack," she says. "I know it sounds stupid, but the kids still need sneakers whether or not their mother has asthma."

"You have to fight the bureaucracy, the insurance companies, and the legislators who don't want to listen. Nobody knows what a financial nightmare this is."

But delaying care also has a price. If she does not keep her migraines under control with medication, she has to go to the hospital emergency room for a Demerol shot. Sometimes she needs the shot even if she has taken her medication. Each emergency room visit costs $64, and she has had six so far this year.

The 20-percent copayments that their Blue Alliance plan does not cover get added to the Winslows' pile of unpaid bills.

"You grow up, get married, have children, get life insurance and health insurance, then someone gets sick," says Deb. "You have to fight the bureaucracy, the insurance companies, and the legislators who don't want to listen. Nobody knows what a financial nightmare this is."

Canada: A well-cushioned safety net.

The Schofields of Wolfville, Nova Scotia, have an 8-year-old son, Matthew, who has tuberous sclerosis, a rare brain disease characterized by mood swings, scizures, tumors on organs of his body, and skin rashes. He wears diapers and functions like a 4- or 5-year-old. Since his illness was diagnosed two years ago, Matthew has been hospitalized three times and made some 40 visits to his family doctor and various specialists.

Nova Scotia's provincial health plan has paid for all that care. In fact, the Schofields have never seen a bill. They simply present their health card, and the hospitals and doctors bill the insurance plan. "We take our medical system for granted," says Matthew's mother, Deanna. "If we had to pay for doctors I don't know what we'd do." Curtis, Matthew's father, is a self-employed carpenter who earns the equivalent of about $12,200 in U.S. dollars.

For about a year after Matthew's illness was diagnosed, the family sometimes went without food and other necessities so they could pay for Matthew's prescription drugs, which cost some $1,300 a year. Nova Scotia's insurance plan does not cover drugs for people under 65. The Schofields tried to get Matthew a policy from Blue Cross (in Canada, Blue Cross can insure services the provincial plans do not cover). But, as in the United States, Canadian Blue Cross organizations accept no one with a severe pre-existing illness.

The local Rotary Club now pays for Matthew's medications. Every time he needs a prescription, the pharmacy automatically bills the club—no claim forms, reimbursements, or money paid out of pocket. The cost of drugs for other family members, some $360 last year, does come out of pocket. But because the province pays their doctor and hospital bills, those expenses are manageable.

Adrianne, Matthew's 6-year-old sister, is susceptible to ear infections and needs antibiotics that cost about $21 each time she is sick. Deanna suffers from urinary-tract infections and kidney stones and often needs antibiotics, too. A few years ago she had to have her kidney stones broken up with a lithotripter. One of Canada's lithotripters is located in Halifax, and Deanna waited three months for treatment. She did not mind the wait. "I was amazed I got in so soon," she says. "If it's an emergency, you get in right away. My stones weren't going anywhere, so there was no urgency to get me in." Until her procedure could be performed, doctors prescribed medication. "I'd rather have waited than have had surgery," she says, referring to the alternative treatment for kidney stones. The provincial insurance plan paid for all her treatment.

Besides bills for prescriptions, the family's only uncovered medical expenses are those for Deanna's and Curtis's dental care. The provincial plan covers dental treatment for children under 12. The family gets additional help from the provincial Department of Community Services, which pays for Matthew's diapers, special soaps and creams, and the family's

---

"They try to keep families together. They know how stressful this is."

---

transportation to Halifax when they take him to doctors there. The Schofields see a family counselor, and the insurance plan pays for those visits. Says Deanna: "They try to keep families together. They know how stressful this is."

OLDER ADULTS WITH HEALTH PROBLEMS

United States: Delayed treatment, greater costs. Tudi Baskay of Alameda, California is 63—too young for Medicare, too poor to buy her own health insurance, and too unhealthy to qualify for it anyway. She is also too typical of women in her age group who have lost their health coverage as a result of a spouse's death or a divorce.

After her divorce in 1990, Baskay had health insurance through COBRA, the federal law that lets divorced people retain their former spouses' insurance coverage for three years. She paid $650 each quarter to Blue Cross of California. But when Blue Cross raised the price to $1,435, she dropped the insurance and tried to get a cheaper Blue Cross plan with fewer benefits. After investigating her health for three months, Blue Cross turned her down. Past medical problems made her ineligible for even a second-rate policy and left her with a stack of unpaid bills.

"I have a choice: Do I relicense my car or have a doctor look at my foot?"

Baskay lives on a 28-foot sailboat. Her annual income of about $13,000 comes partly from her ex-husband's pension and partly from organizing other people's files and closets. That barely covers her dock-space rent and living expenses. "My general health is going to hell because at $90 a pop I can't afford to go to the doctor," Baskay says. "I have a choice: Do I relicense my car or have a doctor look at my foot? You delay everything as long as you can."

Baskay and the U.S. health care system have paid for that delay. A few years ago, she had surgery to correct a minor problem with incontinence, but complications led to a buildup of calcium stones in her urethra. Baskay didn't have $1,200 for the necessary surgery, so her doctor referred her to a county hospital that cares primarily for indigents. Baskay had to wait three and a half months for an examination. Four days after the exam, in pain and unable to walk or urinate, she landed in the emergency room. By the time she had surgery, 10 days later, the stones had grown so large they had to be removed through an incision in her abdominal wall. "I had a totally unnecessary operation—which *was* necessary by the time I had it," Baskay says.

The hospital charged Baskay about $400 of the $542 it cost to treat her before surgery. Her county's "medical services plan," which pays for some care needed by poor people, picked up the $922 hospital tab for her operation.

Her bladder condition has improved, but other medical needs go unmet. This winter she had bronchitis, but "home-dosed" herself with an antibiotic left over from 1988. She says she could not afford to pay for new medicine because she needed to go to the dentist for work on a tooth that was crumbling.

Her vision is blurred, but she has gone without a thorough eye exam for three years. There is a sore on her toe. Is it a fungus or a symptom of something serious? she wonders. Should the spur on her foot be X-rayed? "It's the frustration of being afraid to call my doctor," she says. "I don't like asking for charity. I don't like it one damn bit."

Canada: Quick diagnosis, prompt care.

Joan Brooks, a 58-year-old grandmother, lives in Toronto. Her husband died a year and a half ago after suffering from cancer and kidney failure. He spent his last nine months in the hospital. The Ontario Health Insurance Plan covered all his medical expenses, leaving her no unpaid bills.

Brooks's only income is her husband's veteran's

pension—about $15,000 in U.S. dollars. Paying for medical care is not one of her worries. The Ontario health plan, to which every Ontarian belongs, covers those expenses.

She has severe arthritis and gout in both ankles and is unable to walk unless she takes prescription medicine. Not long ago, she was experiencing dizziness; her doctor suspected a drug toxicity affecting her liver and ordered a diagnostic ultrasound procedure. Brooks had the procedure within one week. She says it could have been done sooner, but her schedule didn't permit an earlier appointment.

When the ultrasound revealed an enlarged liver, her doctor referred her to a specialist. Within days, the specialist admitted her to the hospital's outpatient unit and performed a needle biopsy. The Ontario plan paid the doctor about $54 for his work. Under the rules of the Canada Health Act, the doctor must accept the plan's payment, which is negotiated by the province and the provincial medical association. He cannot bill Brooks any additional amount.

Across Lake Ontario, in Buffalo, New York, insurance carriers pay doctors about $139 to perform the same procedure, and doctors can "balance bill"—that is, charge their patients more than they receive from insurers.

The biopsy showed that Brooks was suffering from excessive fat in her liver. "I'm too fond of the youthful diet," she says. "I have to lose 38 pounds." Her doctor has referred her to a nutritionist at the hospital who is helping her plan low-fat menus.

Right now she takes a drug for arthritis that costs $18 a month. The Ontario plan does not cover prescription drugs for Ontario residents unless they are over 65 or on welfare, but many employed people have drug coverage through private insurance provided by their employers. Brooks has drug coverage because Canada has a number of benefits for its native populations. She is a "status" Indian, which means she is officially registered with the Canadian government as a member of the MicMac nation.

Because of the medication, Brooks's doctor checks her blood every three months to see if the dosage needs fine-tuning. Ontario's health plan pays for the lab tests. When she needs to have her eyes examined, the plan pays for that checkup as well. The insurance plan covers the cost of one complete eye exam each year. Recently she had to return to the optometrist because the glasses he prescribed were inadequate. The plan also covered the second visit, since it pays for subsequent visits if they are necessary.

Brooks is a citizen of both the United States and Canada, because of an old Indian treaty. But she is not interested in trading in Canadian health care for U.S. treatment. "You can't buy the kindness and caring of this system," she says. "I have no dark tales to tell."

HAWAII: COVERAGE FOR ALL

Hawaii likes to think of itself as the "health state." Compared to mainland residents, Hawaiians have a higher life expectancy, spend less time in hospitals, and bear fewer babies who die during their first year of life. Hawaiians have achieved their enviable health status while spending less on medical care than the rest of the nation. In 1988, Hawaii spent about 8 percent of its gross state product on health services; the nation spent about 11 percent of its gross national product.

Dr. John Lewin, director of the state health department, says that Hawaii's good fortune is the direct result of near-universal health insurance coverage and the state's emphasis on primary and preventive care. While those factors are undoubtedly important, the genetic endowments of its ethnic populations, a warm climate, and a less stressful life-style probably contribute, as well.

How It Works

The cornerstone of Hawaii's health care system is the Prepaid Health Care Act, passed in 1974. The act requires all employers to provide health insurance coverage for their full-time workers. They do not have to cover employees' families, but most employers do, since unemployment is low and businesses must compete for workers. The act mandates minimum coverage—120 hospital days, physicians' services, diagnostic and laboratory services, and maternity benefits. Employers can provide more coverage if they wish.

The act requires insurers to accept all employees, even those with health problems. And because everyone is covered, each insurer's "risk pool" automatically includes both the sick and the well. Insurers do not have to pad their premiums to make up for the fact that sick people are more likely to sign up for insurance, as is the case under a voluntary system.

Insurers also save on administrative expenses, since they do not have to screen would-be policyholders.

Employers must pay at least half the premiums, and a worker's share is limited to 1.5 percent of his or her wages. In the beginning, workers and their employers split the cost 50–50. But as wages and premiums have risen, workers have paid a proportionately smaller share.

To assist businesses that employ fewer than eight people and that might have trouble paying, the law authorized a "premium supplementation fund." The fund has grown from the original $300,000 appropriation to $2.3 million in 18 years. "Small businesses never used it and still don't," says Mario Ramil, a Honolulu lawyer and former fund administrator. Over the years, the fund has spent only $89,000 to pay premiums, and those were owed mostly by mainland firms that had left Hawaii.

Covering the unemployed. In 1989, with

$10 million in seed money from the state legislature, Hawaii's health department established the State Health Insurance Plan (SHIP) to cover its "gap" group—people who are unemployed or who work too few hours to be covered by their employers. Most of the 15,000 Hawaiians on SHIP are poor, but not poor enough to qualify for Medicaid.

Benefits under SHIP are not as comprehensive as those provided under the Prepaid Health Care Act. They encourage primary and preventive care rather than costly inpatient hospital services. Patients are entitled to 12 physician visits each year but only five

237

days of hospitalization. Most Hawaiians insured under SHIP must make a $5 copayment for medical services and pay a monthly premium based on their income. The state subsidizes the rest of their care.

Thanks to the Prepaid Health Care Act, SHIP, and Medicaid, only 2 percent of the population lacks some kind of health coverage, compared with about 14 percent in the United States as a whole. "It doesn't occur to us that we can quit a job and not get health insurance," says Valisa Saunders, who works as a nurse. "It's not on our list of things to worry about."

STRENGTHS OF THE HAWAIIAN SYSTEM

Much of the strength of Hawaii's health care system stems from the negotiating power of two major insurers that cover about 70 percent of the population: the Hawaii Medical Service Association (HMSA), a Blue Cross/Blue Shield organization, and Kaiser Permanente, a traditional HMO with salaried doctors working in health centers. That HMO ranked as the best Kaiser plan in the study of HMOs we reported on in Chapter 3.

"We have oligopolistic insurers," says Richard Dahl, a vice president at the Bank of Hawaii, who heads the Governor's Blue Ribbon Panel looking at health care costs. "To some, oligopoly is a dirty word, but not in this state. It provides a pretty efficient system."

Both insurers offer "community rates" to small employers, which make up about 90 percent of all business in the state. That means the insurers charge any group in a community the same rate, no matter what the health experience of a particular group of employees has been. That saves the administrative cost of tailoring individual premiums for particular groups.

"To some, oligopoly is a dirty word, but not in this state. It provides a pretty efficient system."

Because of their large market shares, HMSA and Kaiser have been able to exert some control over health care costs. HMSA has limited fee increases to doctors, paying only cost-of-living raises, and it has begun to eliminate the extra costs imposed by the "unbundling" of physicians' services. (Unbundling means that instead of charging one price for an appendectomy, for example, doctors charge separately for making the incision and removing the appendix.) HMSA now pays doctors one fee for a particular procedure. While some doctors are displeased, there is little they can do. If they participate in HMSA's program, they have to accept the fee. If they do not participate, HMSA simply pays the patients, and the doctors then have to try to collect from them.

The major reason Hawaii's health costs are lower is that Hawaiians spend far fewer days in hospitals than people on the mainland do. Historically, Hawaiians never used many hospital services, having grown up with a system of plantation medicine based on outpatient clinics.

239

HMSA also has designed its insurance policies to favor outpatient and preventive care. With few exceptions, HMSA policies have no deductibles; that encourages people to seek medical attention early, before their conditions worsen to the point at which hospitalization might be required. Policies also pay the minimum rate for a stay in a hospital ward, not the higher semiprivate room rates that mainland insurers typically pay.

Hawaii has not needed a lot of hospitals, so it has not built them. There is little excess capacity. The 28 hospitals on the islands are 80 to 90 percent full.

The question of technology. Hawaii has tried to control medical technology to avoid duplication and waste. It has a health-planning agency and a certificate-of-need law (which requires hospitals and other providers to show why more beds or new medical equipment are necessary before buying them).

The state's health-planning agency has approved seven magnetic resonance imaging machines (MRIs), but did not approve another six that providers asked for. That saved some $15 million in capital costs and almost $13 million a year in operating costs, expenses that undoubtedly would have been passed along in higher premiums.

The state has one lithotripter, which planners say is sufficient to serve the population. Two hospitals had tried to get approval for a lithotripter, but when it was obvious the planning agency would allow only one, they agreed to run it jointly. The lithotripter is now run by a consortium of three hospitals.

WEAKNESSES IN THE HAWAIIAN SYSTEM

Hawaii's health care system is far from perfect. Its problems mirror those found in other states. Most hospitals are having a tough time keeping up with costs. Any efficiencies arising from filled beds, shared services, and low marketing expenses are nearly wiped out by the costs of new technology and medical wage inflation (nurses recently won a 28-percent salary increase over three years). An even greater problem is the failure of Medicare and Medicaid to pay adequately for services used by their beneficiaries.

Medicaid's rolls in Hawaii have swelled by 12,000 people in the last couple of years as eligibility has expanded. The reimbursements to hospitals, however, do not cover the cost of providing care to Medicaid patients. The average daily cost of hospital care in Hawaii (including room, board, and ancillary services) is about $1,000. Medicaid pays only $820. Hospitals charge more for patients with private insurance to cover the shortfall.

The average hospital charge to the two insurers is about $1,500 a day, 50 percent more than the cost. "Cost shifting is going to eat us alive if something isn't done," says HMSA's president, Marvin Hall. Meanwhile, the insurers pass along those extra costs in higher premiums.

Even with its low reimbursements to hospitals, Medicaid is running a serious deficit. This year it required a $64-million emergency appropriation from the state legislature. Next year the program is

241

projected to run $34 million short.

Hawaii is finding that near-universal health insurance coverage is not the same thing as universal care. "There's truly a difference between being eligible for care and actually using the system." says Geri Marullo, deputy director of the state health department. Despite a system of state-funded clinics, medical services are simply unavailable in some areas. Again, the culprit is an underfinanced Medicaid program. On the island of Molokai, for instance, only one physician will treat Medicaid patients. On the Big Island of Hawaii, many dentists refuse to serve them. Medicaid reimburses doctors and dentists only 60 percent of their customary fees, apparently an insufficient amount to persuade providers to care for people who are poor.

As more people become eligible for SHIP and Medicaid, the demands on Hawaii's system inevitably increase. Hawaiians who have always had insurance seem to be using more services, too, a phenomenon partly fueled by the availability of new treatments. Though the state has placed some limits on technology, it may still have too much, says HMSA's president, Marvin Hall. For instance, he thinks Hawaii could make do with three, not seven, MRI machines.

As in other states, some employers have begun to shift part of the increasing cost of health care to their workers in the form of higher copayments. In the pineapple industry, workers now pay $20 for the first visit to a doctor; they once paid $1.

Though there has been some grumbling over higher premiums, no one is seriously talking about scrapping the system Hawaiians have so carefully built. Elise Mastronardo runs an art gallery in a remote corner of the Big Island and pays $6,000 a year in premiums for herself and three employees. "Providing health insurance is not a problem," she says. "It's a cost, but that's all. It's a good thing for people to have."

Lessons learned. Hawaii stands alone among the states in requiring employers to furnish health insurance for their workers. It provides universal insurance coverage, though not necessarily universal access to care. It has also demonstrated that the technological appetite of the medical system, a main driver of health care costs, can be curbed by certificate-of-need laws and planning; and that a limited number of big payers (in this case, one large Blue Cross/Blue Shield organization and one large HMO) can exert some control over the fees of providers.

But Hawaii's clearest lesson may be an unintended one: the pernicious effects of cost shifting when public insurance and private insurance exist side by side. As long as the government can pay less and shift the cost to private insurers, and as long as private insurers can pass the costs on in the form of higher premiums, the crisis in health care will continue.

MINNESOTA'S HMO EXPERIMENT

Half the people in Minneapolis belong to health maintenance organizations. That high concentration

243

of HMO membership makes the Minnesota city a laboratory for managed-care approaches to the health care crisis. According to managed-care theory, HMOs can deliver care more efficiently than traditional fee-for-service medicine. Given a choice, the theory goes, patients will choose the mode of practice that provides the best care at the lowest price.

THE BATTLE AGAINST COSTS

The HMOs' major accomplishment in Minneapolis has been to wring out excess hospital capacity. Twenty years ago, the area had 40 hospitals; today roughly half that number remain. That reduction is the by-product of the hard bargains the HMOs drove in the early years, when they forced the city's hospitals to give them sizable discounts.

The HMOs also found that many hospital inpatient services could be performed as effectively and less expensively in outpatient settings. As HMO members began to use fewer hospital services so, coincidentally, did people who did not belong to HMOs. Doctors in traditional practices learned from the HMO experience that they need not hospitalize as many patients. In the past 18 years, the use of hospital inpatient services has dropped about 50 percent.

The combination of lower fees and fewer patients bankrupted a number of hospitals and forced others to merge. The merger wave, ironically, has left Minneapolis with four hospital systems that are now strong enough to face down the HMOs. "The leverage we have in contracting with hospitals is not as great as it was five years ago. It's more difficult to

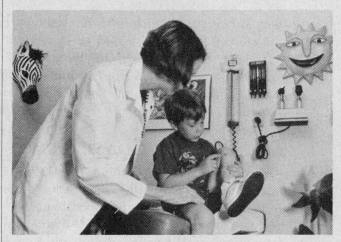

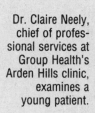

Dr. Claire Neely, chief of professional services at Group Health's Arden Hills clinic, examines a young patient.

negotiate effective rates," says Allan Chernov, medical director of Medica, a large HMO.

HMOs feel the same cost pressures that vex traditional health insurers. HMO premiums have risen as much as 18 percent over the past year, members are using more medical services, drug prices are up, and costly new technology is proliferating as rapidly among HMOs as it is everywhere else. Consider autologous bone-marrow transplants, a procedure for cancer patients that sometimes costs as much as $200,000. In 1990, the city had 40 hospital beds available for that procedure. By 1994, it is expected to have 100. The University of Minnesota Medical Center, which did 200 transplants in 1990, is expected to do twice that many by the end of the decade.

It's hard to say whether that increased capacity is too little, just enough, or too much, since no planning agency exists to evaluate such procedures. This year, Minnesota came close to reinstating a certificate-of-need law, which would have imposed some control over high technology and the number of hospital beds. But opposition from doctors and hospitals defeated that provision in the law that the state finally adopted.

THE ROLE OF CONSUMERS

After 20 years of competition, the HMOs of Minneapolis seem to satisfy their members about equally well. Among those we rated (see Chapter 3), none stood out as better than another. Our survey respondents were equally satisfied with the four largest plans: Physicians Health Plan (now Medica Choice), Group Health, MedCenters, and Share (now Medica Primary). However, only Physicians Health Plan received an above-average rating for member satisfaction with the choice of, and access to, medical specialists.

That HMO allows members to go to specialists whenever they want, without first getting approval from a primary-care physician, as most HMOs require. It also pays its doctors fees for their services, which makes the plan the most expensive one in the Twin Cities. Nevertheless, it has become the biggest HMO in the area, with 330,000 members, or some 60,000 more than its largest competitor. Employers and employees appear willing to pay higher prices for the freedom to go to any doctor.

Some employers have begun to reduce the range of HMO choices for their workers, as a way of eliminating administrative costs. They may, for instance, give employees a choice of one HMO with an option of going outside the plan for care, or an HMO and a preferred-provider organization, all sponsored by the same carrier. As the choices narrow, the consumer has less of a role in selecting the best health plan.

HMOs in Minnesota do virtually all their business with large employers. As a result, they have been no more successful at expanding health care coverage to the 300,000 uninsured people in the state than commercial insurance companies have. They have also shown little interest in signing up consumers who are not part of employer groups, especially people who may be sick. Group Health, for instance, rejected one-quarter of the 4,000 individual applications it received last year.

Even though Minnesota has better coverage for its uninsured citizens than most other states do, their plight had grown severe enough that this year the state set up a program to cover some of them. Even with the new arrangement, the state expects that about 150,000 people still will be without any type of health insurance coverage.

7

TIME FOR
A CHANGE: HEALTH
COVERAGE FOR
ALL AMERICANS

*"It will not be easy to achieve a
single-payer system in the
United States, for the health
industry has much to lose."*

When Dr. James Todd, executive vice president of the American Medical Association, recently met with the editors of *Consumer Reports*, we found ourselves in agreement on the need for reforming the U.S. health care system and even on the principal goals of any reform: universal access to health care, cost control, and improved quality of care. Not surprisingly, however, the AMA, hospitals, and insurance companies can envision only those changes that would touch them least.

Doctors want everyone covered by health insurance but reject the idea of limitations on their fees. "The payer has no right to tell providers what they should charge," Todd said. The American Hospital Association wants to eliminate excess hospital capacity, but it opposes proposals for publicly set budgets that might accomplish just that. Insurance companies want to constrain provider fees, but they do not want to lose the right to sell insurance policies or to pick and choose the Americans they are willing to insure. Businesses want their employees covered by health insurance; they just want to pay less of the bill.

PROPOSALS APLENTY

All these groups embrace managed-care techniques, such as health maintenance organizations, as representing the change least likely to disturb business as usual. In theory, managed care can control provider fees and attempt to improve quality of medical care, even if in practice the record has been spotty at best. But managed care does not address the need to make care available to the uninsured or to reduce the administrative waste and complexity inherent in the present system.

Managed care has become big business, with firms competing fiercely to sell employers the latest money-saving tool. One firm told Consumers Union that it was looking to its next product: how-to manuals that would help people diagnose their own illnesses.

Other reform proposals acknowledge that more

people need insurance coverage, and they would create various mechanisms for accomplishing that end. "Pay or play," the reform backed by some Democrats in the Senate, would require all employers to provide coverage for their workers. If they choose not to "play"—that is, insure their employees—they would have to pay into a special government fund that would supply the coverage. That approach appears to be losing support.

The Bush Administration proposes tax credits to help low-income people buy their own insurance. Health insurers back "small-group reform" that would make it somewhat easier for small businesses to obtain insurance coverage for their employees; so far, 17 states have passed such laws.

All this tinkering around the edges would add some people not now covered to the private insurance rolls. But, as the profiles of the Americans in Chapter 6 demonstrate, owning an insurance policy does not guarantee access to the care you need or make the care you get affordable.

To cover people that insurance companies still do not want or who are too poor to buy insurance even with tax credits, insurance companies and their political allies propose expanding Medicaid, the joint federal and state program to provide health care to the poor. Of course, this solution shifts to the taxpayer the full burden of paying for people whom private insurers find too unprofitable to cover. Since taxpayers will be reluctant to pay higher taxes at the same time that they must pay higher premiums to cover their own families, Medicaid will lack the budgets needed to reimburse providers fairly. As Hawaii's experience shows, when the public portion of the partnership does not pay its share, providers simply charge the private partner more. The Hawaiian experience also shows that Medicaid patients often lack the care they need because some doctors refuse to accept Medicaid's low reimbursement rates.

THE SINGLE-PAYER SOLUTION

A single-payer system that draws its inspiration from Canada's is not the best solution for those doctors who are mainly concerned about their own pocketbooks, or for hospitals with ambitions to become major medical centers. It is certainly a poor solution for health insurance companies; many of them would go out of business. But it is the best solution for the growing number of consumers shut out of the private insurance market and the even larger number who have, with justification, reason to fear that their coverage might disappear at any time. Here's why:

1. A single-payer system eliminates the need for private insurance coverage for basic, medically necessary treatment. The problems with private insurance detailed in Chapters 2 and 5 would instantly disappear. If the United States were to adopt the principles of the Canada Health Act—universality, portability, accessibility, comprehensiveness, and public administration—there would be no need for anyone to buy private insurance policies to cover necessary care. The money

currently spent on insurance premiums and government health programs (Medicare, Medicaid, grants to states) could be redirected to make coverage available for everyone under a single, publicly financed insurance plan.

2. A single-payer system furthers the goal of cost containment by giving a single, influential payer the power to negotiate provider fees and to assure the orderly introduction of technology. Providers would no longer be able to, in effect, dictate their own prices, nor to direct care preferentially at the well-insured while denying it to others, as demonstrated in Chapter 1.

3. A single-payer system allows the payer to experiment with managed-care techniques, collect data, and measure what works and what does not.

4. A single-payer system eliminates the cost shifting to businesses and consumers that results when the government underpays for medical services. Since a single-payer system covers everyone, young and old, rich and poor, there are no private payers to shift to.

It will not be easy to achieve a single-payer system in the United States, for the health industry has much to lose if such a system is adopted, and it is waging a well-financed war against real reform. Its public relations campaigns capitalize on distrust of the government and on the fear of "socialized medicine."

A Model in Medicare

Similar mistrust and fear was used against Medicare before it became law in 1965. Yet the program has been, by most measures, a success. Today Medicare enjoys strong support from the people it serves, while maintaining remarkably low administrative costs, about 2.5 percent of its total expenditures, compared with 4 to 12 percent for private insurance. To administer Medicare, the government employs Blue Cross/Blue Shield organizations and other insurers, which process patients' claims and pay their bills.

The Medicare system has given all elderly people the security of health insurance, a security they lacked before 1965. But it is not without flaws. Among them are the practice of balance billing, which allows doctors to charge patients more than Medicare pays; the complex payment schemes that both patients and providers must cope with; and the gaps in coverage, which have encouraged a bewildering variety of supplemental policies for the elderly. A strong single payer would have the leverage to correct those problems.

As the U.S. health care crisis deepens, and as the medical insecurity of the American people becomes more severe, Consumers Union believes the single-payer approach will make more sense to more people. Then the goals of universal health care, cost control, and quality may at long last become a reality.

APPENDIX
EIGHT WAYS YOU CAN HELP RESOLVE
THE HEALTH CARE CRISIS

A single-payer system of health care guarantees universal access to comprehensive, quality health care at a price that Americans can afford. A single-payer system would eliminate red tape and administrative waste by replacing the current network of 1,500 different insurance companies with a single insurance plan. All health care payments would be made from one source, with overall state and national spending limits, so that total costs could be controlled.

If you agree that Americans deserve a single-payer solution to the national health care crisis, here are eight things you can do right away:

1. *Contact members of Congress to let them know where you stand.*

Write one or more letters to express your support for single-payer health insurance.

✓ Write to your member of Congress in the U.S. House of Representatives. The address is: U.S. House of Representatives, Washington, DC 20515.

✓ Write to your two Senators. The address is: U.S. Senate, Washington, DC 20510.

✓ Send a copy of your letters to: Program for Economic Justice, Consumers Union, 101 Truman Avenue, Yonkers, NY 10703.

✓ Call both Senators and Representatives at: (202) 224-3121.

2. *Contact your governor and state legislators.*

✓ Write letters to your governor and state legislators in support of the single-payer solution. If you don't know where to write, contact your county elections bureau, your local public library, or the League of Women Voters.

3. *Contact candidates for office.*

1992 is an election year.

✓ Before the election, contact candidates for state and federal office and ask them where they stand on single-payer health insurance.

✓ After the election, educate new political officeholders. They may not even be aware that single-payer health insurance is a real option for Americans.

✓ Remember to thank elected officials who do the right thing.

4. Register and vote.

✓ Your views matter! Hold elected officials accountable by making their positions on health care issues an important factor in your voting.

5. Stay informed.

✓ Read newspaper and magazine articles about health care issues. Contact local, state, and national organizations that are working to reform the health care system.

✓ Be skeptical about what you read or hear. Be aware that there are powerful insurance and health care provider groups that oppose single-payer health insurance. These groups are spending lots of money to influence your views.

✓ If criticism of the Canadian system or single-payer is coming from groups representing health care providers or the insurance industry, take it with a grain of salt. Work with others to blow the whistle on misinformation about health care reform. Contact the organizations listed below.

6. Talk back to the news media.

✓ Write a letter to the editor of your local newspaper saying that you support the single-payer solution. Give reasons and facts supporting your position.

✓ Call radio talk shows to express your views.

7.   *Educate others. Create a community dialogue about the need for health care reform and the single-payer solution.*

Virtually every person and every organization in the United States is affected by the health care crisis in some way.

✓ You can help educate others by encouraging community and civic organizations to discuss single-payer health insurance in their programs, panels, and discussion groups.

✓ Arrange for speakers and slide-show presentations for community meetings. To find speakers near you, contact one of the organizations listed on p. 259.

✓ Share this book with a family member or friend.

✓ Make copies of fact sheets on single-payer health insurance and post them in public places. To obtain a sample fact sheet, write to: Program for Economic Justice, Consumers Union, 101 Truman Avenue, Yonkers, NY 10703. Enclose a stamped self-addressed envelope.

8.   *Join organizations working for universal access to health care and single-payer health insurance.*

Dozens of consumer organizations, labor unions, and professional groups support the single-payer concept.

✓ To obtain further information about who supports single-payer health insurance in Congress and the state legislatures, and to learn about new ideas for promoting the single-payer solution, write to the organizations listed below. Ask them if there's a state or local organization near you that can use your volunteer help.

National organizations:

Fund for Health Security
1120 19th Street NW, Suite 630
Washington, DC 20036

Action for Universal Health Care
c/o Northeast Ohio Coalition
for National Health Care
1800 Euclid Avenue, Suite 318
Cleveland, OH 44115

In Texas and New Mexico, contact:

Consumers Union
Southwest Regional Office
1300 Guadalupe, Suite 100
Austin, TX 78701

In California, contact:

Consumers Union
West Coast Regional Office
1535 Mission Street
San Francisco, CA 94103

INDEX

accident policies, 86
activities of daily living (ADLs), 160–61
Aetna, 112, 183
Alzheimer's disease, 161
American Hospital Association, 250
American Integrity, 174, 175, 178
American Medical Association, 249–50
American Republic, 116
American Sun, 183
AMEX Life, 173, 177–78
angiograms, 28
Arizona, 30, 159
assets of old people
   protection of, 153–54, 173–74
   reduction of, 151–53
association groups, 189
atherosclerotic plaque removal, 14–15
AV-MED, 144, 145

back surgery, 15, 54
balloon angioplasty, 24, 26
Bay State Health Care, 119
Blue Cross / Blue Shield of Kentucky, 65–66
Blue Cross / Blue Shield of Massachusetts, 119
Blue Cross / Blue Shield organizations
   administrative costs, 47, 254
   competition with commercial insurers, 65, 67–68
   enrollment policies, 65–68, 78–79
   financial stability, 185
   history of, 7, 66–68
   reimbursement policies, 74
bone-marrow transplantation, 205–6
breast cancer, 60
Bush administration, 197, 206, 251

CAC-Ramsay, 144, 145
California, 45, 84, 143
Canadian health care system, 6, 32, 47, 48, 195–235
   and American system, compared, 220–35
   case histories, 220–35
   costs, 200, 207–8, 213–14, 216–19
   critics of, 196, 215–20
   fees, 198–200
   hospitals, 200–201
   long-term care, 209–12

To order additional copies of *How to Resolve the Health Care Crisis*, use the order form below.

ORDER FORM

CODE	BOOK TITLE (PLEASE PRINT CLEARLY)	QTY.	PRICE EA.	TOTAL
2564P	How to Resolve the Health Care Crisis		$4.95	$

Shipping and Handling:

Orders up to $25 (shipped book rate in U.S.)	$2.50	▶ SHIPPING & HANDLING $
Orders $25.01–$35 (shipped book rate in U.S.)	$3.50	
Orders $35.01 or more (shipped book rate in U.S.)	FREE	
UPS orders (any value) in continental U.S.	$5.00	TOTAL $
Canadian and International orders (any value)	$5.00 (U.S. funds only)	

Name _____

Address _____

City _____ State _____ Zip _____

Payment: Please make check or money order payable to Consumer Reports Books. Allow 2–4 weeks for delivery.

Please charge my credit card.

_____ Mastercard _____ VISA

Card No. _ _ _ _ - _ _ _ _ - _ _ _ _ - _ _

Signature: _____

Mail to: Consumer Reports Books, 9180 LeSaint Drive, Fairfield, OH 45014-5452.

For information on special sales only (10 copies or more), please call Consumer Reports Books at (914) 378-2630, or write to Consumer Reports Books, *How to Resolve the Health Care Crisis*, 101 Truman Avenue, Yonkers, NY 10703-1057.

AFBJA